617.771

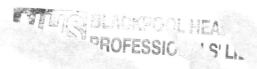

EYELID MYOCLONIA WITH ABSENCES

Dedication

We dedicate this volume to the memory of our friend and colleague Professor Anita Harding whose memorial service was held on 27th November 1995, the day of the symposium from which this book has emanated.

EYELID MYOCLONIA WITH ABSENCES

Edited by

John S. Duncan, MA, DM, FRCP &
C.P. Panayiotopoulos, MD, PhD

John Libbey

JL

LONDON · PARIS · ROME · SYDNEY

British Library Cataloguing in Publication Data

Eyelid myoclonia with absences
1. Eyelids – Diseases
I. Title II. Panayiotopoulos, C.
617.7'71

ISBN: 0 86196 5507

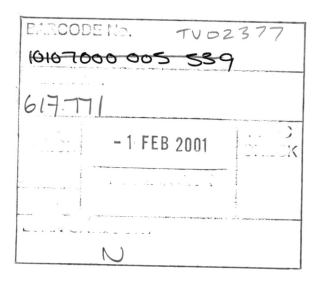
Published by

John Libbey & Company Ltd, 13 Smiths Yard, Summerley Street, London, SW18 4HR, England
Telephone: 0181–947 2777 Fax: 0181–947 2664
John Libbey Eurotext Ltd, 127 Avenue de la République, 92120 Montrouge, France
John Libbey - C.I.C. s.r.l., via Lazzaro Spallanzani 11, 00161 Rome, Italy
John Libbey & Company Pty Ltd, Level 10, 15/17 Young Street, Sydney, NSW, 2000, Australia

© 1996 John Libbey & Company Ltd. All rights reserved.
Unauthorised duplication contravenes applicable laws.

Printed in Great Britain by Thanet Press Ltd, Union Crescent, Margate, Kent, CT9 1NU.
Cover based on a design by S. Sharpe.

CONTENTS

Preface

In 1993 we recognized the need to review current knowledge and controversies relating to typical absences and related epileptic syndromes and organized a conference on this topic in June 1994. This was very successful and led to publication of the volume *Typical Absences and Related Epileptic Syndromes*[1]. There were many areas of controversy in this congress and prominent amongst them was the classification of different syndromes falling within the rubric of idiopathic generalized epilepsy. The syndrome of eyelid myoclonia with absences proved to be of particular interest and this led us to address this topic in detail. Accordingly, we arranged a symposium that was held on the 27th November 1995 at the Royal Society of Medicine in London that was kindly supported by an unrestricted educational grant from Parke-Davis Research Laboratories. The meeting was stimulating and controversial. Manuscripts were also prepared shortly afterwards to reflect current knowledge on this fascinating syndrome and indicate areas of ongoing controversy and fruitful topics for future research.

The book starts with a review of the anatomy and physiology of the eyelids, followed by Professor Jeavons' account of historical aspects. This is followed by discussion of the symptom and the syndromes of eyelid myoclonia with absences, in children and adults. There is then a detailed examination of the controversial area of self induction of absences by eyelid flickering and other mechanisms. The book closes with an account of what is known and not known about the genetics of the condition and strategies for its treatment.

The syndrome of eyelid myoclonia with absences was initially described by Professor Peter Jeavons in 1977. In recognition of this the editors propose that the syndrome of eyelid myoclonia with absences may also be regarded as Jeavons' syndrome.

John S. Duncan
Institute of Neurology,
National Hospital for Neurology
and Neurosurgery
London, WC1N 3BG, UK

C.P. Panayiotopoulos
Consultant in Clinical
Neurophysiology and Epilepsies
St Thomas' Hospital,
London, SE1 7EH, UK

July, 1996

---

1 *Typical absences and related epileptic syndromes (1995), editors, J.S. Duncan & C.P. Panayiotopoulos. London: Churchill Livingstone.*

Eyelid Myoclonia with Absences, edited by J.S. Duncan and C.P. Panayiotopoulos
© 1996 John Libbey & Company Ltd, pp. 1–11.

Chapter 1

Anatomy and physiology of the eyelids

Gordon T. Plant

The National Hospital for Neurology and Neurosurgery, Queen Square, London, WC1N 3BG and Moorfields Eye Hospital, City Road, London, EC1V 2PD

What the eyelids do could not be simpler: they open and close. However, this limited repertoire belies the complexity of the behavioural requirements of the eyelids. They must protect the eye and especially the cornea, and therefore eyelid closure is involved in a number of reflexes with visuosensory and somatosensory afferents. In addition to this, eyelid closure is generated to protect against corneal damage and drying by spontaneous or automatic blinking. In order to remain in a position which is an efficient compromise between corneal protection and unobstructed vision the eyelids must change position in synchrony with vertical eye movements and therefore a range of synkineses is found in relation to ocular motor control and this aspect of the neural control of the lids has features in common with the control of eye movements. The eyelids are also under 'vegetative' control of the sympathetic nervous system, and eyelid position is modulated by autonomic functions regulating, for example, arousal. Eye opening and closure are also intimately concerned with facial expression which is also under both voluntary and involuntary control.

Thus we have a simple movement which is under voluntary, automatic, reflex, emotional and autonomic control. It is not surprising then that abnormalities of eye closure are to be found across the gamut of neurological disorders, from the cerebral cortex to disorders of the muscle fibres. In the following review I have attempted to give something of the flavour of the complexity of eyelid function and dysfunction.

William Gowers (1879) was fascinated by the range of functions of the eyelids and made an early contribution to the importance of understanding the actions of the lids in health and disease (Fig. 1). He appreciated that the eye muscles, the obicularis and the levator, acted together (Fig. 2) and that the voluntary and involuntary movements of the eyelids could be dissociated in disease (Fig. 3). His own drawings here illustrate two patients with chronic partial third nerve pareses and abnormal lid-ocular motor synkineses. When the patient looks downward (second panel) inhibition of the levator should occur but on the left side it is synkinetic *activation* of the levator with the inferior rectus (Fig. 2). However, in voluntary eye closure (third panel) the levator is inhibited synkinetically with the obicularis activation quite normally and symmetrically. The origin of this

1

THE MOVEMENTS OF THE EYELIDS.

BY

W. R. GOWERS, M.D., F.R.C.P.,

ASSISTANT PROFESSOR OF CLINICAL MEDICINE IN UNIVERSITY COLLEGE.

(Received February 11th—Read June 10th, 1879.)

THE movement of the eyelids, and the mechanism by which it is effected, have received very little systematic attention. In the following attempt to explain them it has been necessary to state some familiar facts in order to describe clearly other facts which are not commonly recognised.

Fig. 1. Gowers' classic article on the eyelids (Gowers, 1879).

		Looking down.	Closing eyelids.	
			Gently.	Forcibly.
Orbicularis	. .	No action	... Contraction	... Contraction
Levator	. .	Relaxation	... Relaxation	... Relaxation
Superior rectus.	.	Relaxation	... Inaction	... Contraction
Inferior rectus .	.	Contraction	... Inaction	... Relaxation.

Fig. 2. Gowers' table illustrating the various physiological synkineses between the levator, obicularis and the vertical recti (from Gowers, 1879).

abnormal synkinesis in chronic oculomotor neuropathies is still uncertain (Ezra *et al.*, 1996) more than a century following Gower's first description.

The involuntary movement that is under discussion in this volume is characterized as a form of myoclonus. Myoclonus may be defined as a brief involuntary muscle contraction and indeed many of the earliest descriptions of myoclonus are to be found in descriptions of epileptic phenomena. Unverricht applied the term 'myoklonie' to brief jerks observed in patients suffering from the disorder which today would be called familial myoclonic epilepsy (Unverricht, 1895). Following the description by Jeavons (1977) eyelid myoclonia with absences (EMA) has been distinguished from other epileptic syndromes with myoclonic manifestations. Myoclonus in general may be classified in accordance with the site of generation in the nervous system and a major distinction is between cortical and subcortical myoclonus. Some forms of epileptic myoclonus such as that occurring in epilepsia partialis continua are certainly cortical in origin, as can be shown from back-averaging of the EEG (Thomas *et al.*, 1977). The myoclonus seen in generalized epilepsy is usually considered to be sub-cortical in origin, although direct confirmation of this is lacking and difficult to obtain.

2

Eyelid opening and position

The levator palpebrae superioris is responsible for opening the eyelid and tonically maintains its position. It attaches with the superior rectus to the lesser wing of the sphenoid above the optic foramen, it is a straplike muscle which passes forward below the orbital roof to end in an aponeurotic attachment which fans out across the width of the upper lid. It is innervated by branches of the superior division of the oculomotor nerve (as is the superior rectus). The levator contains only singly-innervated fibres adapted for fatigue-resistant tonic activity (Spencer & Porter, 1988). The fibres are 30–50 microns in diameter and the muscle lacks the extremely small fibres found in the recti (Kuwabara *et al.*, 1975). Müller's muscle consists of smooth muscle fibres and is innervated by the oculosympathetic pathway; the fibres originate from attachments to the striated fibres of the levator and pass forward to insert close to the margin of the upper lid. The frontalis can also elevate the lid because of its attachments with the orbital portion of the obicularis muscle at the eyebrow and this is an important action of the frontalis muscle in patients with ptosis (frontalis overaction).

The control of levator tonic activity is strongly influenced by arousal. Slight lid retraction is a sign of alertness and attention or of anxiety; while we are all familiar with the involuntary inhibition of the levator that occurs as we become drowsy this becomes impossible to overcome voluntarily in extreme fatigue. Gay *et al.* (1967) pointed out that Hering's law of equal innervation applies to the eyelids and this is why contralateral lid retraction is seen in a patient overcoming unilateral levator weakness. The lid retraction is abolished by occluding the abnormal eye.

Gowers (1879) pointed out the close synergy of action of the levator and the superior rectus muscles in downgaze and their dissociation in forced eye closure: in blinking the levator is inhibited, in forced lid closure the levator is inhibited and the superior rectus is activated (Bell's phenomenon; Figs. 2 and 4). He also appreciated that voluntary action is limited and it is not possible to overcome fully the inhibition of the levator which occurs on downgaze. Björk & Kugelberg (1953) published electromyographic recordings showing the relationship between levator tonus and vertical eye position. Ticho (1971) demonstrated a number of synkineses between the levator and *horizontal* eye movements, these showing great individual variability. The levator may

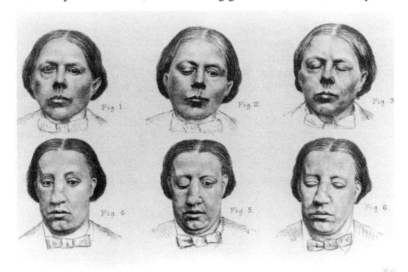

Fig. 3. Gowers' illustration of two cases of chronic partial third nerve paresis showing pathological synkinesis between downgaze and the left levator palpebrae superioris (from Gowers, 1879).

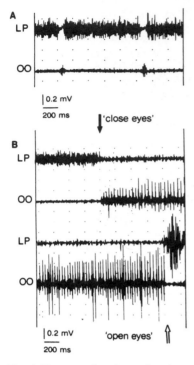

Fig. 4. The normal reciprocal action of levator and obicularis (from Aramideh et al., 1994b).
LP = levator palpebrae;
OO = obicularis oculi

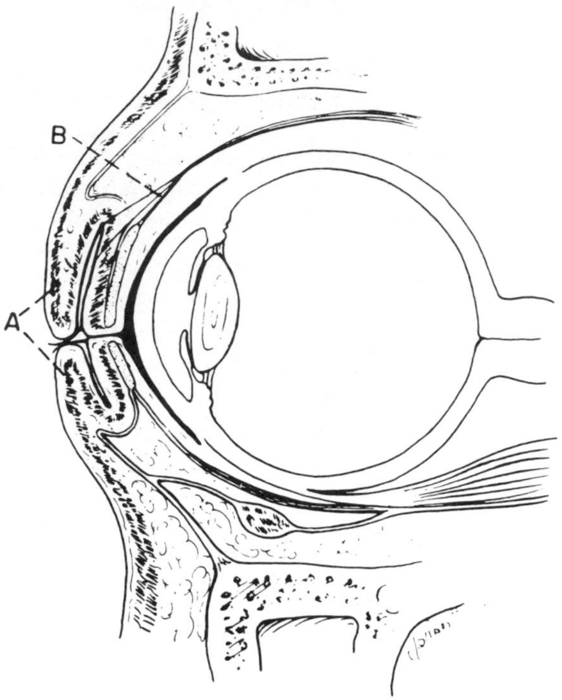

Fig. 5. Schematic vertical section through the eye and lids to show the orbital fibres of the obicularis oculi (A) acting in forced closure of the eyelids. The lashes are buried and the integrity of the palpebral portion of the muscle (see Fig. 6) is maintained by the action of the levator (B) (from Jones, 1961).

be involved in a variety of other facial movements as an associated movement, especially in mouth opening and closure. A variety of pathological synkineses have been described, the best known being the Marcus Gunn jaw winking phenomenon (Gunn, 1883), and Carmichael & Critchley (1925) described a number of physiological synkineses between the eyes and face.

Ptosis and lid retraction are important physical signs. Lid retraction usually results from overaction of the Müller's muscle, as in thyrotoxicosis, or to limited upgaze, because increased activity in the elevators of the eye, whether as a result of weakness of those muscles or restriction caused by fibrosis of the inferior rectus as in dysthyroid eye disease, will result in overaction of the levator muscle if it is not itself weak. Schmidtke & Büttner-Evenner (1992) have recently pointed out that lid retraction in posterior commissure lesions – Collier's sign (Collier, 1927) – is the most commonly observed lid dysfunction of premotor origin.

Eyelid closure

The obicularis oculi is responsible for closure of the eyelids, in sychrony with levator inhibition, and also for movements associated with facial expression. The muscle is composed of three distinct fibre groups: pretarsal, preseptal (together the palpebral portion), and orbital fibres (Figs. 5 & 6). The innermost (pretarsal) fibres are concerned with blinking while the preseptal fibres are concerned with sustained narrowing of the palpebral fissures, and in maximal contraction the eyelashes are buried by the preseptal portion (Fig. 5). Motor units in platysma average 25 fibres (Feinstein *et*

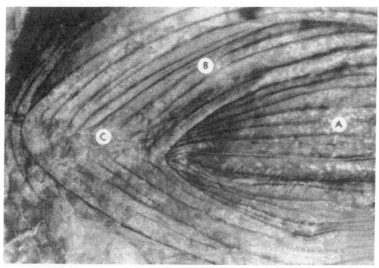

*Fig. 6. The two components of the palpebral portion of the obicularis oculi
muscle are shown in a dissection, the pretarsal (A) and preseptal (B)
portions. The lateral attachment of the preseptal portion is shown at the
lateral palpebral raphé (C) (from Jones, 1961).*

al. 1954) and are thus smaller than most voluntary muscles but larger than motor units in the extraocular muscles. The obicularis oculi is supplied by the facial nerve, from its temporal and zygomatic branches and as the action of the obicularis is to narrow the palpebral fissure it is widened slightly in a facial palsy.

Gordon (1951) carried out a classic study in which he recorded the activity of motor units in his own left eyelid. He was aware of the existence of the functional subdivisions between different anatomical regions of the obicularis (Fig. 6) and found that blinks, which obscured vision for about 130 ms, were initiated by bursts of high frequency impulses, including double discharges, lasting about 55 ms. Very high firing rates (180 s) were found in motor units in the palpebral portion nearest the lids and these units fire only during blinks and it may not be possible to activate them in sustained voluntary contractions (Fig. 7). It did not seem to be possible to grade a blink voluntarily. In weak sustained voluntary contraction low threshold units with relatively low firing

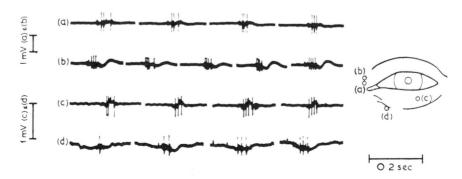

*Fig. 7. Motor unit activity recorded from the pretarsal portion of the obicularis oculi muscle
during involuntary blinking (from Gordon, 1951).*

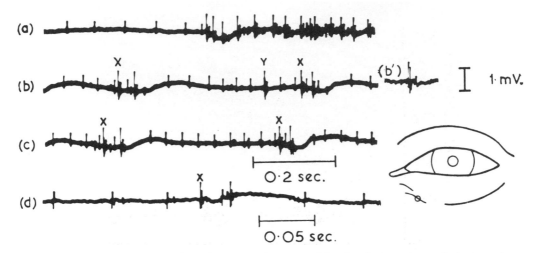

Fig. 8. Motor unit activity recorded from the preseptal portion of the obicularis oculi muscle during voluntary eye closure (from Gordon, 1951).

rates (50 impulses/s) which are located away from the lid margins are recruited (Fig. 8). Some units in the outer margins of the lids which showed relatively low impulse frequencies during blinking were also activated in unilateral winking and stronger graded voluntary contraction. In maximal voluntary contractions activity is seen in units in the outer (orbital) regions of the obicularis. Fibres of the lower lid are not involved in blinking and show recruitment on upward gaze. The location of the mechanism which coordinates the levator and obicularis synchrony is not known (Fig. 4). There is no reciprocal activity during unilateral voluntary winking (Cogan, 1956).

It has been known for many years that blinks are generated synchronously with saccades (Hall, 1945). Blinks during saccade shifts have recently been investigated by Evinger et al. (1994). Some patients with abnormally slow saccades can generate normal saccades coincident with a blink (for example, Huntington's disease). Periodic blinks, as well as being related to eye movements, are modulated by attention and emotional factors. Parkinsonism reduces spontaneous blink frequency and elevated dopaminergic stimulation increases it (see Karson, 1984). Complex reflex activity involving eye closure is associated with yawning, laughing, crying and sucking.

In a study of eye closure evoked by cortical stimulation in primates Leyton & Sherrington (1917) made the important observation that the cortical fields which evoked eyelid opening and closure were widely separate. They were also studying limb, hand and other movements and in most other cases reciprocal movements were evoked by stimulation of adjacent points. Eye closure (bilateral except close to threshold) was achieved by stimulation of the precentral gyrus close to the hand area, whereas eye opening was more likely to be seen following stimulation of occipital or frontal cortex anterior to the precentral gyrus and almost always occurred in association with conjugate movements of the eyes. These fields for eye opening tended to be somewhat more diffuse. Subsequently eyelid closure has been shown to occur following stimulation of mesial temporal lobe, amygdala and cingulate gyrus in human and primate, all independently of motor cortex integrity. The eyelid closure that follows stimulation of the amygdala is ipsilateral and follows facial and jaw movements. The afterdischarge, if bilateral, is associated with bilateral eye closure and chewing movements (Baldwin et al. 1954). Eyelid flutter and forced rapid blinking have been described in occipital epilepsy (for example, Gastaut, 1960) and reproduced by electrical stimulation (Penfield & Jasper, 1954).

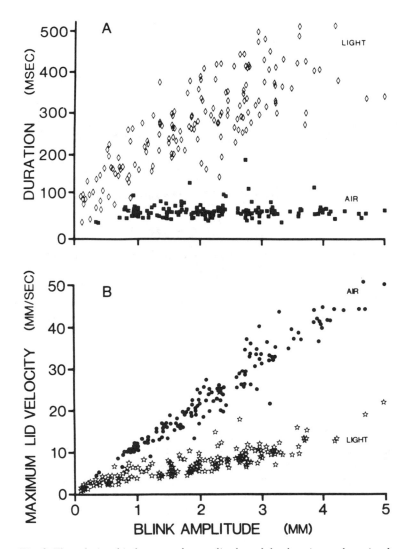

Fig. 9. The relationship between the amplitude and the duration and maximal velocity of blinks evoked either by light or corneal stimulation in the rabbit (from Manning & Evinger, 1986).

Reflex control of the obicularis oculi

Levinsohn (1913) was one of the first to distinguish the variety of reflexes involving blinking. Blink reflexes have served as a model for behavioural learning, for example associative learning (McCormick & Thompson, 1984) and reflex modification (Hoffman & Ison, 1980). A monosynaptic stretch reflex can be recorded from the obicularis oculi and the corneal blink reflex is of course very familiar; blinks and blepharospasm can also be elicited by acoustic stimulation.

In reflex blinking it is possible to identify an immediate *preprogrammed* activity which is followed by a *stimulus dependent* component. This was shown clearly by Manning & Evinger

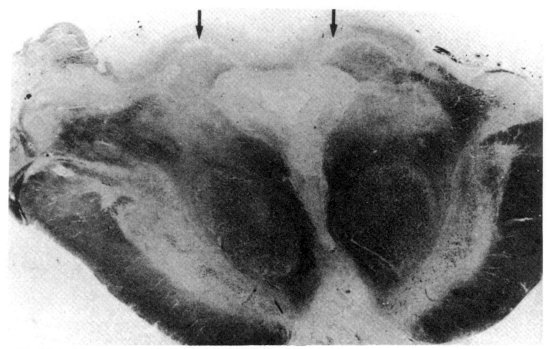

Fig. 10. In the case reported by Tavy et al. (1984) the light evoked blink reflex was preserved in a patient in whom the cerebral cortex was severely damaged and the superior colliculi (arrow) were necrosed.

(1986) studying blinks in the rabbit evoked either by light or corneal air puffs. In this study the differences between blinks evoked by corneal stimulation as opposed to light were shown to have different characteristics; the former are extremely brief yet achieving amplitudes as great as or greater than the slower light-evoked blinks (Fig. 9).

The light stimulus evoked blink reflex appears to be mediated by optic nerve fibres that pass to the superior colliculus and pretectal region. Keane (1979) provided good evidence that the blink response to light is a brain stem reflex in a patient who had intact blink reflex to light but no optokinetic nystagmus or blink to visual threat. At necropsy there was complete necrosis of all the cerebral cortex. In a similar case described by Tavy *et al.* (1984) the superior colliculi were also necrosed, indicating that the pretectal area may be responsible for the reflex (Fig. 10). Rushworth (1962) showed adaptation if the stimulus is at regular intervals but not if randomly presented. Startle blinks have a longer latency (80 ms) than light evoked blinks (50 ms). The reflex blink to visual threat probably does require an intact cortex (Liu & Ronthal 1992).

Blepharospasm occurs in response to a variety of stimuli, and severe corneal pain provokes reflex blepharospasm which is the cause of the 'blindness' in 'snow blindness'. Apart from the piste this was also a common occurrence in the days when tram lines were repaired late at night using oxyacetyline blowpipes: casual observers, perhaps on their way home from a public house, would appear in the hospital casualty department believing themselves to be blinded until a few drops of local anaesthetic were applied to each cornea. In essential blepharospasm, repeated involuntary forceful closure of the eyelids in which orbital, preseptal and pretarsal portions all contribute occurs. Blepharospasm is also seen in Meiges syndrome, tardive dyskinesia, neurodegenerations, and brainstem lesions (Jancovic & Patel, 1983). The occurrence of blepharospasm in brain stem lesions (Jancovic & Patel, 1983) and abnormalities of the blink reflex have led to the suggestion that blepharospasm is a type of focal dystonia resulting from abnormal brain stem function. Aramideh *et al.* (1994a) have shown that involuntary eyelid closure may involve only the obicularis, may involve involuntary inhibition of the levator, disturbed reciprocal innervation of the two muscles, or finally levator inhibition alone. This latter disorder has been called 'apraxia' of eyelid opening (Goldstein & Cogan, 1965) although Schmidtke & Büttner-Ennever (1992) have stated that the term should be abandoned because the executive motor system is affected in this disorder. Usually the eyes reopen normally after a blink.

Involuntary eye movements are also found in association with essential blepharospasm. Aramideh *et al.*, (1994b) have shown recordings of these movements and have suggested that they are akin to 'oculogyric crises', that is to say a dystonic form of eye movement, possibly generated in the brain stem. They consisted principally of upward deviation of the eyes and it is difficult to distinguish all such movements with certainty from Bell's phenomenon occurring synkinetically with eye closure which is sometimes seen to persist following treatment of blepharospasm with botulinum toxin (Elston, 1992). However, synkinetic eye and dystonic limb movements have also been reported (Paine, M., Riordan-Eva, P., Plant, G.T., *unpublished*).

The term blepharoclonus had been used to indicate brief rhythmic contractions of the obicularis oculi (Behrman & Scott, 1988). It is usually elicited on gentle eye closure (occasionally on eye opening (Obeso *et al.*, 1985); in extrapyramidal disease it may be seen in isolated blepharospasm and in other extrapyramidal disorders with or without associated blepharospasm. It has also been described as a gaze-evoked phenomenon in multiple sclerosis (Carmichael & Critchley, 1925; Keane, 1978). 'Fluttering' of the eyelids is also seen in normal individuals as a tic-like phenomenon.

Conclusion

This review has drawn from the complexity of the known physiology information which may be relevant to the great variety of paroxysmal eye closure phenomena in epilepsy. The paroxysmal activity underlying these phenomena, which could be arising in a number of cortical or subcortical locations, is usually unknown. A detailed study of the associated levator, facial and ocular motor activity in the paroxysms may provide additional insight into the mechanisms involved. Similarly the relationship between eye closure and paroxysmal EEG abnormalities in some patients is not well understood. Eye closure alone (in darkness) and abrupt onset of darkness without eye closure are not effective in causing paroxysmal EEG discharges, indicating a synergy between the act of eye closure and reduction in illumination. As can be seen above there are a number of pathways whereby eye closure can be achieved and a systematic study of the relative importance of these in inducing paroxysmal activity could be useful.

References

Aramideh, M., Ongerboer, de Visser, B.W., Koelman, J.H.T.M., Bour, L.J., Devriese, P.P. & Speelman, J.D. (1994a): Clinical and electromyographic features of levator palpebrae superioris muscle dysfunction in involuntary eyelid closure. *Mov. Disord.* **9**, 395–402.

Aramideh, M., Bour, L.J., Koelman, J.H.T.M., Speelman, J.D. & Ongerboer de Visser, B.W. (1994b): Abnormal eye movements in blepharospasm and involuntary levator palpebrae inhibition: clinical and pathophysiological considerations. *Brain* **117**, 1457–1474.

Baldwin, M., Frost, L.L., Wood, C.D. (1954): Investigation of primate amygdala: movements of the face and jaws. *Neurology* **4**, 586–598.

Behrman, S., Scott, D.F. (1988): Blepharoclonus provoked by voluntary eye closure. *Mov. Disord.* **3**, 326–328.

Björk, A. Kugelberg, E. (1953): The electrical activity of the muscles of the eye and eyelids in various positions and during movement. *Electroencephalogr. Clin. Neurophysiol.* **5**, 595–602.

Carmichael, E.A., Critchley, M. (1925): The relationship between eye movements and other cranial muscles *Br. J. Ophthalmol.* **9**, 49–52.

Cogan, D.G. (1956): *Neurology of the ocular muscles.* pp. 139–148, 2nd edition, Springfield, Illinois: Charles C. Thomas.

Collier. J. (1927): Nuclear ophthalmoplegia: With especial reference to retraction of the lids and to lesions of the posterior commisure. *Brain* **50,** 488–498.

Elston, J.S. (1992): A new variant of blepharospasm. *J. Neurol. Neurosurg. Psychiatry* **55,** 369–371.

Evinger, C, Manning, K.A., Pellegrini, J.J., Basso, M.A., Powers & A., Sibony, P. (1994): Not looking while leaping; the linkage of blinking and saccadic gaze shifts. *Exp. Brain Res.* **100,** 337–344.

Ezra, E., Spalton, D., Sanders, M.D., Graham, E.M., Plant, G.T. (1996): Ocular neuromyotonia. *B. J. Ophthalmol.* **80,** 350–355.

Feinstein, B. Lindegård, B., Nyman, E & Wohlfart, G. (1954): Morphological studies of motor units in normal human muscles. *Acta Anat.* **23,** 127–142.

Gastaut, H. (1960): Un aspect meconnu des decharges neuroniques occipitales: la crise oculo-cloniques ou 'nystagmus épileptique'. In: Alajouanine Ed *Les Grands Activités du lobe Occipital.* Paris: Masson et Cie. pp. 169–185.

Gay, A.J., Salmon, M.L., Windsor, C.E. (1967): Hering's law, the levators and their relationship in disease states. (1967): *Arch. Opthalmol.* **77.**

Goldstein, J.E., Cogan, D.G. (1965): Apraxia of lid opening. *Arch. Opthalmol.* **73,** 155–159.

Gordon, G. (1951): Observations upon the movements of the eyelids. *B. J. Ophthalmol.* **35,** 339–351.

Gowers, W.R. (1879): The movements of the eyelids. *Medico-Chirurgical Transactions* **62,**429–440.

Gunn, R.M. (1883): Congenital ptosis with peculiar associated movements of the affected lid. *Trans. Ophthalmol. Soc. UK* **3,** 283–287.

Hall, A. (1945): The origin and purposes of blinking. *B. J. Ophthalmol.* **29,** 445–467.

Hoffman, H.S. & Ison J.R. (1980): Reflex modification in the domain of startle. I. Some empirical findings and their implications for how the nervous system processes sensory input. *Psychol. Rev.* **87,** 775–189.

Jancovic, J., Patel, S.C. (1983): Blepharospasm associated with brainstem lesions. *Neurology* **33,** 1237–1240.

Jeavons, P.M. (1977): Nosological problems of myoclonic epilepsies in childhood and adolescence. *Dev. Med. Child Neurol.* **19,** 38.

Jones, L.T. (1961): An anatomical appproach to problems of the eyelids and lacrimal apparatus. *Arch. Ophthalmol.* **66,** 111–124.

Karson, C.N., Burns, R.S., LeWitt, P.A., Foster, N.L., Newman, R.P. (1984): Blink rates and disorders of movement. *Neurology* **34,** 677–678.

Keane, J.R. (1978): Gaze-evoked blepharoclonus. *Ann. Neurol.* **3,** 243–245.

Keane, J.R. (1979): Blinking to sudden illumination: a brainstem reflex present in neocortical death. *Arch. Neurol.* **36,** 52–53.

Kuwabara, T, Cogan D.G., Johnson, C.C. (1975): Structure of the muscles of the upper eyelid. *Arch. Ophthalmol.* **93,** 1189–1197.

Levinsohn, G. (1913): Der optische Blinkrefles. *Z. Gesamte Neurol. Psychiatr.* **20,** 377–385.

Leyton, A.S.F. Sherrington, C.S. (1917): Observations of the excitable cortex of the chimpanzee, orang-utan and gorilla. *Q. J. Exp. Physiol.* **11,** 135–222.

Liu, G.T. & Ronthal, M. (1992): Reflex blink to visual threat. *J. Clin. Neuroophthalmol.* **12,** 47–56.

Manning, K.A., Evinger, C. (1986): Different forms of blinks and their two stage control. *Exp. Br. Res.* **64,** 579–588.

McCormick, D.A., Thompson, R.F. (1984): Cerebellum: essential involvement in the classically conditioned eyelid response. *Science* **223,** 296–299.

Obeso, J.A, Artieda, J., Marsden, C.D. (1985): Stretch reflex blepharospasm. *Neurology* **35,** 1378–1380.

Penfield, W. & Jasper, H. (1954): *Epilepsy and the functional neuroanatomy of the human brain.* London: Churchill.

Rushworth, G. (1962): Observations on blink reflexes. *J. Neurol. Neurosurg. Psychiatry* **25,** 93–108.

Schmidtke, K, Büttner-Ennever, J.A. (1992): Nervous control of eyelid function: a review of clinical and experimental data. *Brain* **115,** 227–247.

Spencer, R.F., Porter, J.D. (1989): Neuroanatomy of the oculomotor system. Structural organisation of the oculomotor system. Editor: J.A. Büttner-Ennever. Amsterdam: Elsevier, pp. 33–79.

Tavy, D.L.J., van Woerkom, T.C.A.M., Bots, G.T.A.M. & Endtz, L.J. (1984): Persistence of the blink reflex to sudden illumination in a comatose patient: a clinical and pathologic study. *Arch. Neurol.* **41**, 323–324.

Thomas, J.E., Regan, R.J., Klass, D.W. (1977): Epilepsia partialis continua. *Arch. Neurol.* **34**, 266–275.

Ticho, U. (1971): Synkinesis of upper lid elevation occurring in horizontal eye movements. *Acta. Ophthalmol.* **49**, 232–238.

Unverricht, H. (1895): Über familiäre Myoklonie. *Deutsche Zeitschrift für Nervenheilkunde.* **7**, 32–67.

Eyelid Myoclonia with Absences, edited by J.S. Duncan and C.P. Panayiotopoulos
© 1996 John Libbey & Company Ltd, pp. 13–15.

Chapter 2

Eyelid myoclonia and absences: the history of the syndrome

P.M. Jeavons

Aston University, Aston Triangle, Birmingham, B4 7ET, UK

The original description of this form of photosensitive epilepsy (Jeavons, 1977) was based primarily on clinical findings, confirmed by EEG. It seems best to quote the original paragraph:

'Eyelid myoclonia and absences show a marked jerking of the eyelids immediately after eye closure and there is an associated brief bilateral spike and wave activity. The eyelid movement is like rapid blinking and the eyes deviate upwards, in contrast to the very slight flicker of eyelids which may be seen in a typical absence in which the eyes look straight ahead. Brief absences may occur spontaneously and are accompanied by 3 cycles per second spike and wave discharges. The spike and wave discharges seen immediately after eye closure do not occur in the dark. Their presence in the routine EEG is a very reliable warning that abnormality will be evoked by photic stimulation.'

The eyelid movements are very obvious and can be seen at a distance – parents often regard them as tics. The associated discharge of spike and wave or polyspike and wave occurs within 3 seconds of eye closure and does not last longer than 3 or 4 seconds. Persistent spike and wave activity is not seen.

In 1982 a change in the term from eyelid myoclonia *and* absences to eyelid myoclonia *with* absences was a mistake (Jeavons, 1982), since it implied that an absence was induced by the eye closure whereas in fact absences occurred independently of the closure, often being induced by hyperventilation. A few patients also had occasional tonic-clonic seizures.

Attacks tend to be worse in bright light and a number of the patients described by Ames (1971; 1974) appeared to have eyelid myoclonia – these patients' attacks are self-induced, as are those described by Darby *et al.* (1980) and Binnie *et al.* (1980). These authors reported patients who carried out a slow eye closure movement which was followed by a spike wave discharge, the diagnosis being made during the course of prolonged EEG recording, which they said was necessary to identify their syndrome. They also commented that eye closure on command did not produce this effect. However, we found eyelid myoclonia commonly occurred in our patients during routine EEG examination. Some, but not all, of our patients with eyelid myoclonia are similar to those described by the above authors. The sex ratio of their 13 patients was approximately 1:1 whilst in our patients 80 per cent are female. This predominance of females is the same as is found in other photosensitive epilepsies. The mean age of onset is around 6 years, similar to that of absences, and earlier than that of other photosensitive epilepsies, which is at 13 to 14 years.

Therapy is less effective than in other photosensitive epilepsies (Covanis *et al.* 1982). Complete control of seizures was achieved in only 63 per cent of 19 patients, compared to 77 per cent in juvenile myoclonic epilepsy with photosensitivity, 76 per cent in pure photosensitive epilepsy, and 87 per cent in absence seizures without photosensitivity. Sodium valproate was the most effective drug but it was necessary to use a higher dose than for other seizures, and some patients required ethosuximide in addition.

Gobbi *et al.* (1985) reported 11 patients, eight being male and three female. Early onset was confirmed, seizures having appeared before the age of 6 years in eight of the patients. There was no true myoclonus of the eyelids on polygraphic recording. The duration of the seizures was between 1 and 3 seconds in seven cases, but one girl showed absence status on eye closure. Although eye closure provoked seizures, blinking did not. In seven cases the discharges appeared between 0.2 and 2 seconds after closure of the eyes but in the remaining four the discharges occurred 2 to 4 seconds after eye closure. These last four patients were photosensitive and the types of seizure varied. Nine of the 11 cases were treated with sodium valproate alone or in combination with ethosuximide, and control was achieved in six. Relapse occurred on withdrawal of medication.

Gobbi *et al.* (1989) found 51 cases in the literature concerning seizures presenting with eye closure, excluding self-induced seizures. They gave details of 24 cases. Continuous myoclonic jerks when the eyes were closed were seen in seven cases, eyelid myoclonia in five, absences in four, atypical absence or absences with a tonic component in three, myoclonic jerks in one, tonic-clonic seizures in one, and three had other or unspecified seizures. They described 22 of their own cases (10 male and 12 female) and 11 had eyelid myoclonus with absences. The remaining 11 were divided into two groups, one consisting of five cases with bilateral myoclonic jerks or absences with myoclonus whilst the other group showed continuous repetitive myoclonic jerks when the eyes were closed and persisting afterwards. This latter group is a type of absence status and it appears probable that eyelid myoclonus should be included in their first group.

Dalla Bernardina *et al.* (1989) described 17 patients with eyelid myoclonus, all but one showing abnormality on intermittent photic stimulation. Seven were regarded as having juvenile myoclonic epilepsy, two had benign myoclonic epilepsy of infancy, two petit mal absences, two had absences and tonic-clonic epilepsy and the remaining four were classified as eyelid myoclonus epilepsy. However, these last differed from those described by Jeavons (1977; 1982) in that their seizures only occurred on eye closure and they did not have absences. Their mean age of onset was 8 years, similar to that of juvenile myoclonic epilepsy. They commented that eyelid myoclonus tended to disappear between the age of 15 and 18 years and concluded that it is an age dependent electro-clinical manifestation. However many other authors have shown that it persists into later adult life. These authors made no comment about self induction and their illustration does not seem to show slow blinking.

Appleton *et al.* (1993) described five cases of eyelid myoclonia with absences, confirming the clinical picture, the early onset, and the efficacy of sodium valproate with or without ethosuximide. These authors did not find evidence of self induction.

Covanis *et al.* (1994) reported on 25 patients, of whom 19 were female, and confirmed an early onset (mean 7 years). All showed spike and wave or polyspike and wave on eye closure and hyperventilation evoked spike and wave in 60 per cent. All patients had photoparoxysmal responses with interrmittent photic stimulation. Seizures were completely controlled in 56 per cent with valproate monotherapy and the addition of lamotrigine controlled two more patients. Relapse occurred in seven patients on withdrawal of medication.

Conclusion

In conclusion a syndrome can be identified on the basis of the clinical manifestations, EEG findings, age of onset, and response to therapy and prognosis. Eyelid myoclonia with absences is a variety of photosensitive epilepsy and although some patients undoubtedly self-induce it is not primarily a syndrome of self induction.

References

Ames, F.R. (1971): Self induction in photosensitive epilepsy. *Brain* **94,** 781–798.

Ames, F.R. (1974): Cine film and EEG recording during 'hand-waving' attacks of an epileptic photosensitive child. *J. Electroencephalogr. Clin. Neurophysiol.* **37,** 301–304.

Appleton, R.E., Panayiotopoulos, C.P., Acomb & B.A., Beirne, M. (1993): Eyelid myoclonia with typical absences: An epilepsy syndrome. *J. Neurol. Neurosurg. Psychiatry* **56,** 1312–1316.

Binnie, C.D., Darby, C.E., De Korte, R.A. & Wilkins, A.J. (1980): Self-induction of epileptic seizures by eye closure: incidence and recognition. *J. Neurol. Psychiatry.* **43,** 386–389.

Covanis, A., Jeavons, P.M. Gupta, A.K & Jeavons, P.M. (1982): Sodium valproate: monotherapy and polytherapy *Epilepsia* **23,** 693–720.

Covanis, A., Skiadas, K., Loli, N., Ioannidou, A. Lada, Ch, & Theodorou, V. (1994): Eyelid myoclonia with absence. *Epilepsia* **35,** (suppl 7.) p. 13 New York: Raven Press.

Dalla Bernadina, B., Sgro, V., Fontana, E., Cellino, M.R., Moser, C., Zullini, E., Grimau-Merino, R. & Blasi-Esposito, S. (1989): Eyelid myoclonia with absences. In: *Reflex Seizures and Reflex Epilepsies:International Symposium on Reflex seizures and Reflex Epilepsies,* eds. A., Gastaut, H., Naquet, R. Beaumanoir. Geneva, June 1988, Geneva Editions Medicine & Hygiene, pp. 193–200.

Darby, C.E., De Korte, R.A., Binnie, C.D. & Wilkins, A.J. (1980): The self-induction of epileptic seizures by eye closure. *Epilepsia* **21,** 31–41.

Gobbi, G., Tinuper, P., Tassinari, C.A., Aguglia, U., Bureau, M., Dravet, C., Roger, J. & Gastaut, H. (1985): Eyelid myoclonia absences. *Bollettino-Lega Italiania Contro L'Epielessia* **51/52,** 225–226.

Gobbi, G., Bruno, L., Mainetti, S., Parmeggiani, A., Tullini, A., Salvi, F., Tassinari, C.A., Santanelli P, Bureau, M., Dravet, C. & Roger, J. (1989): Eye closure seizures. In: *Reflex Seizures and Reflex Epilepsies:International Symposium on Reflex seizures and Reflex Epilepsies,* eds. A., Gastaut, H., Naquet, R. Beaumanoir. Geneva, June 1988, Geneva Editions Medicine & Hygiene, pp. 193–200.

Green, J.B. (1966): Self-induced seizures: clinical and electroencephalographic studies. *Arch. Neurol.* **15,** 579–586.

Jeavons, P.M. (1977): Nosological problems of myoclonic epilepsies in childhood and adolescence. *Dev. Med. Child Neurol.* **19,** 38.

Jeavons, P.M. (1982): In: *Myoclonic epilepsies: therapy and prognosis.* eds. H. Akimoto, H. Kasamatsuri, M. Seino, A. Ward, *Advances in Epileptology: XIIIth Epilepsy International Symposium.* New York: Raven Press, pp. 141–144.

Eyelid Myoclonia with Absences, edited by J.S. Duncan and C.P. Panayiotopoulos
© 1996 John Libbey & Company Ltd, pp. 17–26.

Chapter 3

Eyelid myoclonia with absences: the symptoms

C.P. Panayiotopoulos, A. Agathonikou, M. Koutroumanidis, S. Giannakodimos, S. Rowlinson and C.P. Carr

Department of Clinical Neurophysiology and Epilepsies, St. Thomas' Hospital, London, England

Eyelid myoclonia with absences: the syndrome

Eyelid myoclonia with absences (EMA) is a distinct syndrome of idiopathic generalized epilepsy (IGE) characterised by the triad of eyclid myoclonia associated with brief absences, generalized discharges of 36 Hz polyspikes and slow waves which are brief (usually 3–4 s) precipitated mainly by eye closure and photosensitivity.

As Jeavons (1977) was the first to recognise EMA, it is reasonable to propose that EMA should be named Jeavons syndrome.

It should be emphasized from the outset that EMA is more of a myoclonic (localised in the eyelids) than an absence syndrome. Impairment of consciousness is often mild and the EEG manifestations are mainly of the polyspike type. Eyelid myoclonia should not be confused with the rhythmic or random eyelid closure occurring in typical absences of other epileptic syndromes.

Eyelid myoclonia with absences: the seizure

The hallmark of EMA is eyelid myoclonia, not the absences which are mild and are seen only as part of the eyelid myoclonic seizure (Giannakodimos & Panayiotopoulos, 1996). Eyelid myoclonia is usually the first symptom to attract attention although it is often misinterpreted as a 'tic' or mannerism. Once seen, eyelid myoclonia will never be forgotten.

The seizure of EMA was described by Jeavons (1977) as follows:

'The characteristic seizure is a brief episode of marked jerking of the eyelids with upwards deviation of the eyes, associated with a generalized discharge of spike-wave, and occurring on closure of the eyes.'

However, eyelid myoclonia is often confused with other ictal eyelid manifestations occurring during typical absences in IGE.

The purpose of this study was to describe the ictal clinical manifestations of eyelid myoclonia in patients with EMA and the eyelid and eye ictal manifestations of typical absences in other forms of idiopathic generalized epilepsy.

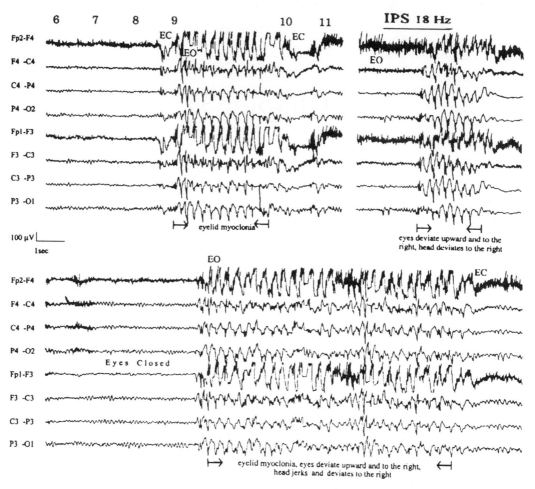

Fig. 1. Video-EEG on awakening after partial sleep deprivation of a 32 year-old female with EMA. She had continuous clusters of seizures in this recording.
Top left: a brief absence occurred on eye closure while the patient was counting. This was associated with eyelid myoclonia and opening of the eyes. An ictal delay in pronouncing the successive number was recorded. Top right: intermittent photic stimulation with the eyes open. This was associated with eyelid myoclonia, rhythmic jerking of the head and deviation of the eyes and head to the right. Bottom: A generalised polyspike/spike and slow wave discharge of 9s duration occurred while the patient had the eyes closed. Half a second after the onset of the discharge, the eyes opened because of rhythmic jerking of the eyelids, eyebrows and head, and the eyes and head deviated to the right. These clinical manifestations lasted until 1 s before the end of the discharge. EC = eye closure, EO = eyes open. (From Giannakodimos & Panayiotopoulos, 1996. With permission from Epilepsia).

We have studied with video-EEG the ictal manifestations during the generalized discharges in 15 patients with strict clinical EEG evidence of EMA (see above definition of the syndrome) and 90 patients with idiopathic generalized epilepsies and video-EEG documented absences.

Video-EEG: ictal clinical and EEG manifestations in Jeavons syndrome

All 15 patients had at least one routine video-EEG and eight had 14 additional video-EEGs during sleep and on awakening. Ictal phenomena were recorded in all but one case who had a normal EEG. The clinico-EEG ictal manifestations of the seizures were as follows:

Eyelid myoclonia with absences. Fig. 1

This most typical type of seizures in EMA occurred in eight patients. The seizure starts with eyelid myoclonia consisting of repetitive, often rhythmic, fast (4–6 Hz), small or large range myoclonic jerks of the eyelids which make the eyes open and close with simultaneous vertical jerking and upwards deviation of the eyeballs. The eyes retain a semi-open position during the ictus irrespective of whether the seizure starts when eyes were closed, open or on eye closure. This is probably due to a coexistent tonic contraction of the eyelid elevators during the seizure. Occasionally, simultaneous jerks of the eyebrows and/or the head could be seen. Eyelid myoclonia was often associated with lateral deviation of the eyes and the head and could be arrhythmic. The eyelid jerks varied in force, amplitude and number between seizures, even in the same patient. Occasionally the eyelid jerks could be single but often there were more than three repetitive jerks. Rarely eyelid myoclonia could be associated with jerks of the hands. In one patient the tonic component of the eyelid semi-opening and the deviation of the eyes and head was more apparent than the associated clonic components. Polyspikes were the predominant EEG accompaniments in this patient.

Absences occurred only as part of this type of eyelid myoclonic seizure and while the eyelid myoclonia continued, although less violently than at the onset. Impairment of consciousness was usually mild, manifested with cessation, repetition, errors and delays of breath counting. Impairment of consciousness was rarely so severe as to prevent the patients recalling phrases given to them during the ictus. Automatisms were never observed.

The EEG ictal accompaniments were generalized discharges of mainly polyspikes and polyspikes slow waves at a frequency of 3–6 Hz (usually more than 4 Hz) and a duration of 3–6 s (usually around 3 s) (Fig. 1). A seizure lasted more than 6 s only once. Polyspikes were more apparent and were often continuous (uninterrupted by slow waves) in the first 1–2 s from onset. Polyspike and slow waves usually followed this multiple spike opening phase of the discharge. The onset of the EEG discharges was simultaneous or preceded the eyelid jerks.

Eyelid myoclonia without absences. Fig. 2

Eyelid myoclonia, often associated with jerks of the eyeballs, head or other muscles as described above but without discernible absences, occurred in all eight patients with eyelid myoclonia and absences and in another six additional patients. The ictal EEG manifestations were generalized mainly polyspike discharges of brief (1–2 s, rarely 3–5 s) duration. Some polyspike and slow wave components could be seen at the end of the discharge.

The same patient with EMA could manifest, in the same or other video-EEG sessions, severe and milder eyelid manifestations consisting of brief (usually less than 1 s, but 1–3 s duration could occur), abortive eyelid myoclonia with eyelid tremor-like jerks or fast eyelid fluttering. In the latter occasions, the eyes remained closed while the upper eyelid showed small range fast fluttering which would be difficult to appreciate without close range video-EEG recordings.

These milder eyelid manifestations could be the only type of seizures in some patients, particularly those relatively well controlled on medication. They were associated with polyspikes in the ictal EEG.

Slow eye-closure could also occur but the EEG discharges, mainly of polyspikes, were apparent before the termination of the eye-closure artefact, probably indicating that the tonic component of the eye-closure was an ictal phenomenon.

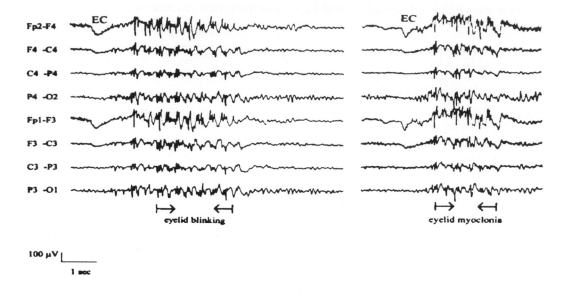

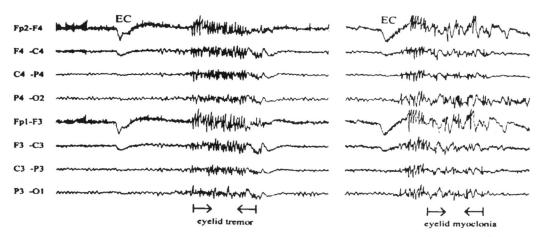

Fig. 2. Four variants of eye closure related abnormalities in a 36-year-old female with EMA (case 9 in Giannakodimos & Panayiotopoulos, 1996).
Top left: 1 s after eye closure a generalized polyspike and slow wave discharge occurs. Note that initially the discharge contains mainly polyspikes. Clinically, the patient shows eyelid blinking that starts 1.5 s after eye closure, and ends with the EEG discharge.
Bottom left: 2 s after eye closure, a 2.5 s generalised discharge of a series of polyspikes at around 12 Hz, associated with eyelid tremor-like movements.
Right (top and bottom): these two eye closure-related discharges, although clinically manifested with identical eyelid myoclonia and upward deviation of the eyes, differ electroencephalographically in that the second one (right bottom) begins with a series of polyspikes lasting for 1 s and not associated with obvious clinical manifestations. EC = eye closure, EO = eyes open.
(From Giannakodimos & Panayiotopoulos, 1996. With permission from Epilepsia).

We have never observed the repetitive eye blink-like movements in ictal absences of EMA and absences never occurred without some form of eyelid myoclonia preceding their onset.

Eyelid and eye movements as ictal manifestations of typical absences

We studied 90 patients with IGE and video-EEG recorded typical absences (> 2.5–3 Hz spike and/or polyspike and slow wave with clinical manifestations).

They all had IGE with absences alone or combined with myoclonic jerks and/or generalized tonic-clonic seizures (GTCS).

Syndromes included: childhood absence epilepsy, juvenile absence epilepsy, myoclonic absence epilepsy, perioral myoclonia with absences, phantom absences with generalized tonic-clonic seizures, absences with single myoclonic jerks and also other unclassified syndromes of idiopathic generalized epilepsy with typical absences (Panayiotopoulos *et al.*, 1995).

Fifty four were female and their age ranged from 2–62 years. Twenty one were 10 years old or younger.

There were 536 recorded typical absences (>2.5–3 Hz spike and/or polyspike and slow wave with clinical manifestations). Each patient had from one to 35 recorded absences (median five absences)

Additional numerous generalized discharges (polyspikes, spike/slow waves) without clinical manifestations could occur and they were more than those associated with clinical manifestations, particularly in adults and during sleep.

Thirty nine (43.3 per cent) of the 90 patients had eyelid or eyes-related ictal clinical manifestations. Opening of the eyes during the absences could occur but it is not included in this study (Panayiotopoulos *et al.*, 1989).

It should be realized that it is extremely difficult to describe and classify movements of the eyelids and eyes. We have tried to simplify things by taking into account the most prominent manifestations although symptoms often overlapped in the same patient and even for the same seizure. We classified them as consistent if they occurred in every absence in the same patient and inconsistent if they were present in some but not all of the absences in the same individual. Symptoms included the following phenomena:

a. Similar to the spontaneously occurring eyeblinks of normal people and they could be random or repetitive and rhythmic during the absence

b. Eyelid fluttering which was similar to the eyelid fluttering occurring in mild forms of eyelid myoclonia

c. Predominantly rhythmic and vertical eyebrow oscillations

d. Vertical and/or rotatory nystagmus

e. Eyelid myoclonia-like symptoms

The following is the best classification we could achieve for the ictal clinical manifestations from the eyelids and eyes during the typical absences of the 90 patients:

- Fourteen patients had inconsistent eyelid blinking during the absence ictus
- Four patients had inconsistent eyelid fluttering
- Six patients had consistent eyelid blinking
- Four patients had consistent eyelid fluttering
- One patient had vertical nystagmus
- Five patients had eyebrow rhythmic movements
- EMA-like ictal manifestations were recorded in five patients

Thus, 39 out of the 90 patients had ictal manifestations from the eyelids and eyes but in only five (5.6 per cent) of them did have these some similarities with those occurring in EMA (Fig. 3). Only one of those five patients was photosensitive, and all but one (Fig. 4) did not have the consistent eye-closure induced abnormalities of EMA.

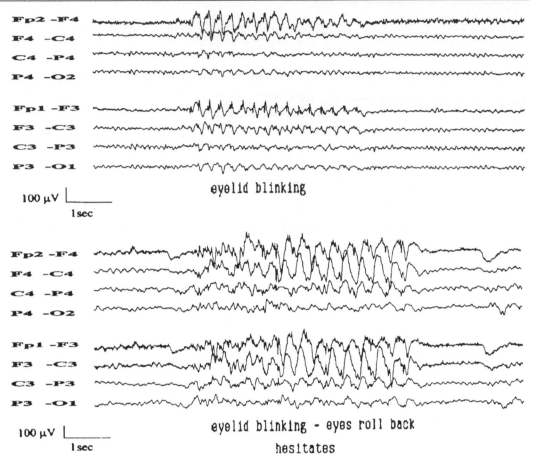

Fp2 –F4
F4 –C4
C4 –P4
P4 –O2

Fp1 –F3
F3 –C3
C3 –P3
P3 –O1

100 μV | ____
1 sec

eyelid blinking

Fp2 –F4
F4 –C4
C4 –P4
P4 –O2

Fp1 –F3
F3 –C3
C3 –P3
P3 –O1

100 μV | ____
1 sec

eyelid blinking - eyes roll back
hesitates

Fig. 3. Upper: Video-EEG of a 33-year-old female who had onset of clinically detectable typical absences with marked eyelid manifestations from the age of 12 to 20 years. She had a single nocturnal GTCS at the age of 14 years. Sodium valproate was discontinued at the age of 25 years. Presently she is not aware of absences. The video-EEG showed frequent spontaneous and overbreathing-induced generalised discharges of high amplitude spike/polyspike and slow wave for up to 5.5 seconds. Some of them were associated with small range eyelid fluttering and in only one of them there was a repetition of the same number during breath counting. She was not photosensitive.
Lower: Video-EEG after partial sleep deprivation of a 12-year-old girl who started having typical absences at the age of 9 years. Absences were resistant to medication with Sodium Valproate. There are frequent generalised discharges of polyspikes and slow waves lasting up to 8 seconds, associated with fast eyelid blinking, semi-opening of the eyes and vertical jerking of the eye balls. There is severe ictal impairment of consciousness. She is not photosensitive.

Photosensitivity amongst 90 patients with absences

Twenty patients (22.2 per cent) had clinical and/or video-EEG documented photosensitivity but only five of them had eyelid and eyes-related ictal clinical manifestations during the absences (Fig. 5).

Two patients had random eyelid blinking which is strikingly different from the eyelid myoclonia of Jeavons syndrome. Two patients had fast rhythmic eyelid fluttering/blinking.

One patient had EMA-like manifestations.

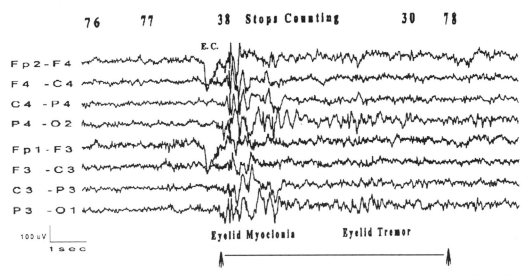

76   77   38 Stops Counting   30   78

Fig. 4. Video-EEG of a 10-year-old girl with brief episodes of eyelid myoclonia and backward jerking of the head from the age of 4 years. These are exaggerated when she is anxious or if she is engaged in solving difficult problems. She is not clinically or EEG photosensitive.
The video-EEG demonstrated eyeclosure discharges. Thirteen out of 23 eyeclosures were followed by generalized discharges which were clinically manifested by eyelid myoclonia, upward tonic or clonic deviation of the eyeballs and occasionally by a single backward jerk of the head. Mild impairment of cognition was always a feature and was manifested by errors in counting.
The clinico-EEG seizure in this figure is of interest because the eyelid myoclonia and the impairment of cognition during the discharge is followed by eyelid tremor-like movements and disturbance of consciousness despite the apparent cessation of the discharge.
The duration of the clinical seizure is indicated with the arrows. Patient was counting (annotated numbers). The discharges were totally inhibited in darkness.

Observations in 'normal' persons

Having studied, with video-EEG recording, the ictal manifestations from the eyes and eyelids of patients with absences, we investigated similar manifestations in normal people. We soon realized that with the exception of the violent myoclonic jerks of the eyelids, all other symptoms could often be manifested by ordinary people we meet in our work or social environment. The eyes and the eyelids are the most sensitive and expressive parts of our body and relevant reviews and reports on the spontaneous and reflex eye blinking, eyelid fluttering and other movements in normal people and patients can be found in textbooks of neuro-ophthalmology (Walsh, 1957) and there is an extensive literature on the subject.

For the purpose of this study we examined a small sample from people appearing on the television (interviews, round table discussions and debates) and we reached the following conclusions:

(1) When under tension, the rate of spontaneous blinks increases significantly. In some people this may become repetitive in clusters of 3–5 s which show close similarities to that described in self-induced photosensitive epilepsy. This type of repetitive blinking was apparent either at the beginning (like a breath before starting a sentence) or at the end of it (like a relief). It was particularly apparent when talking on sensitive matters and was not observed when the same people were not participating in the discussion. It is like tics which are a motor expression of emotional disturbance. Other normal subjects may semiclose their eyelids with brief transient fluttering.

Typical Absenses and Photosensitivity

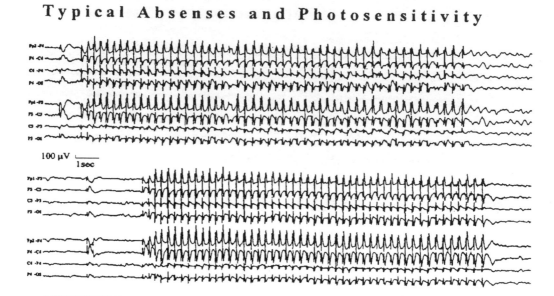

IPS

Fig. 5. Video-EEG of a 9 year-old boy with photically (TV, video-games)-induced seizures during which he complained of headache and might vomit. He becomes 'vacant and not with it'. He also had complex visual hallucinations and fear. In addition, he had typical absences. There is a strong paternal and maternal family history of epileptic disorders. In the video-EEG there is ictal loss of consciousness, de novo automatisms and random or rhythmic eyelid blinking.

(2) Slow and sustained eyeclosure was rarely manifested mainly by women when talking about their distress, anger or frustrations.

(3) Less frequently, eyes were widely opened with cessation of spontaneous blinks.

Therefore, all forms of ictal eyelid and eye movements (except the violent myoclonic jerks of the eyelid myoclonia) occurring in absences can also be expressed in normal people under certain circumstances (Hall, 1936; 1945). We do not know the significance of this, which is a very interesting phenomenon to study which is but beyond the scope of this chapter.

Conclusion

The eyelid myoclonia of EMA is the most frequent and characteristic seizure manifestation which persists in adult life even after absences and other seizures have been controlled by appropriate medication (Panayiotopoulos, 1994a,b;1996a,b; Giannakodimos & Panayiotopoulos, 1996). The full scale eyelid myoclonia of this syndrome is distinctly different from the random or rhythmic eyelid closing or fluttering during the course of typical absences in other epileptic syndromes and the repetitive eye closure attempts for self-induction (see chapter 10)

However, it should also be emphasized that the symptom/seizure of eyelid myoclonia alone is not sufficient to characterize the syndrome of EMA, as it may also be seen infrequently (five out of 90 patients) in other cases of idiopathic generalized epilepsy with absences.

Eyelid myoclonia has also been described in other epileptic conditions, mainly cryptogenic and symptomatic (Panayiotopoulos *et al.*, 1992; 1995; Ferrie *et al.*, 1995; Fish, 1995) and we have described a patient with eyelid myoclonia and fixation-off sensitivity who was not photosensitive and had learning difficulties (Panayiotopoulos, 1987). Similar cases of intractable cryptogenic generalized epilepsy and fixation-off sensitivity have also been described by other authors (Gumnit *et al.,* 1965; Barclay *et al.,* 1993; see for review Panayiotopoulos, 1995a).

Also, early forced eyelid blinking and flutter, myoclonic jerks of the eyelids and oculoclonic activity may occur in occipital sezures, as documented with deep stereo-EEG recordings which may not show in scalp EEG (see review by Williamson *et al.,* 1992). An interesting patient with symptomatic partial seizures consistently induced by deviation of the eyes was reported by Shanzer *et al.* (1965). The partial seizures consisted of unresponsiveness, and 'shimmering, fluttering', rotatory and upward rapid eye movements' followed by turning of the head and clonic movements of the right hand and leg. This lasted for approximately half a minute and was not associated with discernible EEG changes despite interictal focal spikes and slow waves.

Furthermore, the intensity of eyelid myoclonia in EMA may vary from very severe (violent jerks of the eyelids and eyes) to very mild (eyelid fluttering, tremor-like). The latter may be seen in normal people and patients with other absences.

However, it is justifiable to support the view that the symptom of eyelid myoclonia associated with absences is highly suggestive of EMA. It becomes most likely when it is associated with photosensitivity and it is pathognomonic when it also occurs after eye-closure.

There are also other differentiating symptoms such as short duration of absences, mild impairment of consciousness, and mainly polyspikes in the generalized EEG discharges.

Acknowledgements

We thank the Special Trustees of St. Thomas' Hospital for financial support for our studies on the epilepsies.

References

Barclay, C.L., Murphy, W.F., Lee, M.A. & Zarwish, H.Z. (1993): Unusual form of seizures induced by eye closure. *Epilepsia* **34,** 289–290.

Ferrie, C.D., Giannakodimos, S., Robinson, R.O. & Panayiotopoulos, C.P. (1995): Symptomatic typical absence seizures. In: Typical absences and related epileptic syndromes, eds. J.S. Duncan and C.P. Panayiotopoulos, pp. 241–252. London: Churchill Livingstone.

Fish, D.R. (1995): Blank spells that are not typical absences. In: Typical absences and related epileptic syndromes, edited by J.S. Duncan and C.P. Panayiotopoulos, pp. 253–262. London: Churchill Livingstone.

Giannakodimos, S. & Panayiotopoulos, C.P (1996): Eyelid myoclonia with absences in adults: a clinical and video EEG study. *Epilepsia* **37,** 36–44.

Gumnit, R.J., Niedermeyer, E., & Spreen, O. (1965): Seizure activity uniquely inhibited by patterned vision. *Arch. Neurol.* **13,** 363–368.

Hall, A.J. (1936): On the acts of closing and opening of the eyes. *Br. J. Ophthalmol.* **20,** 257–295.

Hall, A.J. (1945): The origin and the purpose of blinking. *Br. J. Ophthalmol.* **29,** 445–467.

Jeavons, P.M. (1977): Nosological problems of myoclonic epilepsies in childhood and adolescence. *Dev. Med. Child. Neurol.* **19,** 38.

Panayiotopoulos, C.P. (1994a): Fixation-off-sensitive epilepsies: clinical and EEG characteristics. In: *Epileptic seizures and syndromes,* ed., P. Wolf, pp. 55-65. London: John Libbey.

Panayiotopoulos, C.P. (1994b): The clinical spectrum of typical absence seizures and absence epilepsies. In: *Idiopathic generalized epilepsies: clinical, experimental and genetic aspects,* eds. A. Malafosse, P. Genton, E. Hirsch, C. Marescaux, D. Broglin, R. Bernasconi R., pp. 75–85. London: John Libbey.

Panayiotopoulos, C.P. (1996a): Fixation-off sensitive, scotosensitive and other visual-related sensitive epilepsies. In: *Reflex epilepsies,* eds. S. Zifkin *et al.* New York: Raven Press (in press).

Panayiotopoulos, C.P. (1996b): Absence epilepsies: childhood, juvenile and myoclonic absence epilepsy, eyelid myoclonia with absences and other related epileptic syndromes with typical absence seizures. In: *Epilepsy: a comprehensive textbook,* eds., J.E. Engel & T.A. Pedley. (Volume 3, in press). New York: Raven Press.

Panayiotopoulos, C.P., Obeid, T. & Wakeed, G. (1992): Differenttiation of typical absences in epileptic syndromes. A video-EEG study of 224 seizures in 20 patients. *Brain* **112,** 1039–1056.

Panayiotopoulos, C.P., Chroni, E., Daskalopoulos, C., Baker, A., Rowlinson, S. & Welsh, P. (1992): Typical absence seizures in adults: clinical, EEG, video-EEG findings and diagnostic/syndromic considerations. *J. Neurol. Neurosurg. Psychiatry* **55**, 1002–1008.

Panayiotopoulos, C.P., Giannakodimos, S. & Chroni, E. (1995): Typical absences in adults. In: *Typical absences and related epileptic syndromes,* edited by J.S. Duncan and C.P. Panayiotopoulos. pp.289–299. London: Churchill Livingstone.

Shanzer, S., April, R. & Atkin, A. (1965): Seizures induced by eye deviation. *Arch. Neurol.* **13**, 621–626.

Walsh, F.B. (1957). *Clinical neuro-ophthalmology.* Second edition. Baltimore: pp. 186–245. The Williams & Wilkins Company.

Williamson, P.D., Thadani, V.M., Darcey, T.M., Spencer, D.D., Spencer, S.S. & Mattson, R.H. (1992): Occipital lobe epilepsy: clinical characteristics, seizure spread patterns. and results of surgery. *Ann. Neurol.* **31**, 313.

Eyelid Myoclonia with Absences, edited by J.S. Duncan and C.P. Panayiotopoulos
© 1996 John Libbey & Company Ltd, pp. 27–31.

Chapter 4

Eyelid myoclonia with absences in children: the Cardiff experience

Sheila J. Wallace

Consultant Paediatric Neurologist, University Hospital of Wales, Heath Park, Cardiff CF4 4XW

Introduction

The analysis of the components of absence seizures by simultaneous video and electroencephalographic (EEG) recordings was pioneered by Penry *et al.* (1975), who described mild clonic components, usually of the eyelids, in 45.5 per cent of 374 absence seizures in 48 patients. Two years later, Jeavons (1977) identified, amongst children presenting with absence seizures, a group in whom, immediately after eye closure, marked jerking of the eyelids occurred, associated with brief bilateral spike-and-wave activity. Deviation of the eyes upwards was also noted. In addition, these children had spontaneous brief absences accompanied by 3 Hz spike-and-wave activity on the EEG. Jeavons (1977) also emphasized that all these children were photosensitive. Eyelid myoclonia with typical absences (EMA) has been more clearly defined by Appleton *et al.* (1993), who argued that this type of epilepsy should be given the status of a separate syndrome.

In this communication I examine the characteristics of 41 children with absence seizures who were seen between 1991 and 1995, inclusive, with a view to determining whether, in circumstances where simultaneous EEG and video recording is not available, those children with eyelid myoclonia and photosensitivity are readily separable from others with absences.

Patients and Methods

Patients were referred to the paediatric neurology service at the University Hospital of Wales either directly from primary care doctors or from general paediatricians. Children with epilepsy with myoclonic absences and those with absences and perioral myoclonia are not included in this report. For the 41 patients identified, the mean duration from the onset of absences to attendance at the paediatric neurology clinic was 1.6 years. Twenty-six of the children had no eyelid myoclonia, and 15 were observed to have myoclonic/clonic movements of the eyelids during absences. Two of the latter 15 are photosensitive and their characteristics are examined separately in the tables. Their case histories are as follows:

Patient 1

A male, was referred by a general paediatrician when aged 5 years. His seizures had started at 2 years of age with frequent episodes of loss of awareness associated with head turning to the left, eyelid jerking, and elevation or deviation to the left of the eyes. His EEG showed bilateral 3 Hz spike-and-wave, with photosensitivity, and occasional phase-reversing right frontal sharp waves. Up to 36 seizures were recorded each day. Therapy with valproate, up to 20 mg/kg/day, produced an incomplete response and the valproate was withdrawn. Carbamazepine had been introduced, with worsening in seizure frequency and increase in the eyelid jerking.

It was recommended that the carbamazepine should be discontinued and that valproate be re-introduced and given at a higher dosage. This child had no first degree relative with seizures, but a maternal aunt suffered from an uncategorized epilepsy. He had had delay in speech development and was struggling to keep up in a mainstream class.

Patient 2

A male, whose mother had had a single febrile seizure as a child, was first seen in the paediatric neurology clinic at the age of 6 years. His teacher was concerned by lapses in awareness. At the age of 3 years, two generalized tonic-clonic seizures had occurred, and some episodes of loss of awareness and jerking had been noted. No EEG was recorded and a general paediatrician prescribed valproate, which was continued until about 6 months before referral to the paediatric neurologist. No seizures were observed while valproate was being given. Overall development, but particularly speech, had been delayed; there were minor difficulties with balance, fine movements, praxis and right-left orientation; and, behaviour was problematical. Education was in mainstream school with specific extra help. Absences were observed to be associated with jerking of the eyelids and a tendency to lean forwards; some perioral jerking was also seen. During a routine EEG, the patient refused to close his eyes or to hyperventilate, but photic stimulation at 18–22 flashes/second, with the eyes open only, evoked bursts of high voltage, 3–4 Hz generalized spike-and-wave, associated with clinical changes. Valproate was reintroduced. A further EEG, at age 9 years, while still receiving valproate, showed no seizure discharges and no evidence of photosensitivity.

The family histories, clinical details, EEG characteristics and responses to therapy for all 41 children with absences are given in tables 1 to 4.

Table 1. Seizures in first degree relatives

Seizure type in relative	Ab n = 26	AbEM n = 13	AbEMP n = 2
Absences	0	*2	0
Febrile seizures	2	2	1
Generalized tonic-clonic	2	*2	0

Ab = no eyelid myoclonia; AbEM = absences with eyelid movements not photosensitive;
AbEMP = eyelid myoclonia + photosensitivity.
* One child had first degree relatives with both absences and generalized tonic-clonic seizures.

Results

Comparison of the children with typical features of eyelid myoclonia and absences with the others was difficult because of the small number involved. Table 1 shows that a history of a seizure disorder in a first degree relative is not a differentiating feature. Table 2 emphasises the very young age of onset but shows that, where eyelid myoclonia and photosensitivity co-exist, other seizures, school placement, neurological findings and behavioural difficulties are not additional differentiating features. As expected, all 41 children had generalized 2.5–3.5 Hz spike-and-wave discharges on their EEG. In addition, three of those who were not observed to have myoclonia involving the eyelids, as well as the two who did, were photosensitive. Twenty patients had EEG abnormalities other than generalized spike-and-wave. When unilateral or bilateral frontal discharges were seen, three-quarters of the patients had eyelid jerking, whereas central or temporal discharges were seen only in those who had no eyelid jerking. Table 4 mainly reflects choices of therapy made by referring doctors. Both the patients with eyelid myoclonia and photosensitivity had some response to valproate, one responding completely, and the other incompletely to a low dose. Inappropriate therapy had been prescribed in six patients.

Table 2. Clinical details

Clinical details	Ab n = 26	AbEM n = 13	AbEMP n = 2
Sex: males	12	6	2
Age onset (years): mean	7.2	7.0	2.5
range	3–13	4–11	2,3
Other seizures	5	1	1
generalized tonic-clonic	4	0	1
febrile seizures	1	1	0
School placement			
mainstream, no extra help	17	10	1
poor progress	5	1	1
good progress	12	9	0
special help in mainstream	7	0	1
special needs unit	2	3	0
Neurological findings			
normal	19	11	1
minimal alterations	2	1	1
dyspraxia	5	1	0
Behavioural problems present	7	2	1

Ab = no eyelid myoclonia; AbEM = absences with eyelid movements present;
AbEMP = eyelid myoclonia + photosensitivity.

Discussion

The importance of simultaneous split-screen video-EEG recordings in the diagnosis of EMA has been emphasized previously (Appleton *et al.* 1993; Appleton, 1995). It is clear that without this facility, cases may be missed. My study examines areas other than photosensitivity through which EMA may be identified. Only the very early age at onset seems an additional pointer. Thus it is important to consider whether failure to diagnose EMA would have untoward consequences. Appleton (1995) suggests that children with EMA do well scholastically, but there is ample evidence from other sources (Binnie *et al.* 1987, Goode *et al.* 1970) that spike-and-wave activity interferes with cognition. Both the boys described above had difficulties in school. Clearly the seizures of EMA should be eliminated, if possible.

The tendency for EMA to persist beyond childhood has been noted on several occasions. Patient 2 had a relapse of his absences when valproate was withdrawn after more than 2 years in apparent remission. Recognition of EMA is likely to lead to more realistic treatment plans and patient counselling.

The relevant criteria for classification of absence epilepsies have been explored in detail by Hirsch *et al.* (1994), who analysed data on 43 patients, who had 570 absences recorded. These authors conclude that, in isolation, eyelid myoclonias are not specific, since they have also been reported in childhood absence and in juvenile myoclonic epilepsy. Photosensitivity with self-stimulation was considered by Hirsch *et al.* (1994) to be the most characteristic feature of EMA.

Table 3. *Electroencephalographic findings*

Electroencephalographic abnormalities	Ab n = 26	AbEM n = 13	AbEMP n = 2
Generalized spike/wave discharges	26	13	2
Focal discharges			
Frontal: bilateral	1	3	0
unilateral	2	5	1
Central/temporal: bilateral	0	0	0
unilateral	8	0	0
Photosensitivity	3	0	2
Seizure induced by computer game	1	0	0

Ab = no eyelid myoclonia; AbEM = absences with eyelid movements present;
AbEMP = eyelid myoclonia + photosensitivity.

Table 4. *Response to treatment*

Drugs used	Ab n = 26	AbEM n = 13	AbEMP n = 2
Treated with ethosuximide	9	9	0
complete control	4	1	0
some response	0	0	0
controlled + 1 other AED	2	1	0
no response	1	4	0
poor compliance, intolerance	2	3	0
Treated with valproate	20	10	2
complete control	9	4	1*
some response	3	2	1
controlled + 1 other AED	3	1	0
no response	2	1	0
no information	1	2	0
poor compliance/intolerance	2	0	0
Other therapy used			
clonazepam	1	1	0
lamotrigine	2	1	0
vigabatrin**	0	1	1
carbamazepine**	3	2	

Ab = no eyelid myoclonia; AbEM = absences with eyelid movements present;
AbEMP = eyelid myoclonia + photosensitivity.
* relapsed after withdrawal of valproate.
**prescribed by general paediatricians before referral to paediatric neurologist.

References

Appleton, R.E. (1995): Eyelid myoclonia with absences. In: *Typical absences and related epileptic syndromes*, eds. J.S. Duncan & C.P. Panayiotopoulos, pp. 213–220. London: Churchill Livingstone.

Appleton, R.E., Panayiotopoulos, C.P., Acomb, B.A. & Beirne, M. (1993): Eyelid myoclonia with typical absences: an epilepsy syndrome. *J. Neurol. Neurosurg. Psychiatry* **56,** 1312–1316.

Binnie, C.D., Kasteleijn-Nolst Trenité, D., Smit, A.M. & Wilkins, A.J. (1987): Interactions of epileptiform EEG discharges and cognition. *Epilepsy Res.* **1,** 239–245.

Goode, D.J., Penry, J.K., Dreifuss, FE. (1970): Effect of paroxysmal spike-wave on continuous visuo-motor performance. *Epilepsia* **11,** 241–254.

Hirsch, E., Blanc-Platier, A. & Marescaux, C. (1994): What are the relevant criteria for a better classification of epileptic syndromes with typical absences? In: *Idiopathic generalized epilepsies: clinical, experimental and genetic aspects,* pp. 87–94, eds. A. Malafosse, P. Genton, E. Hirsch, C. Marescaux, D. Broglin & R. Bernasconi. London: John Libbey.

Jeavons, P.M. (1977): Nosological problems of myoclonic epilepsies in childhood and adolescence. *Dev. Med. Child Neurol.* **19,** 38.

Penry, J.K., Porter, R.J. & Dreifuss, F.E. (1975): Simultaneous recording of absence seizures with videotape and electroencephalography: a study of 374 seizures in 48 patients. *Brain* **98,** 427–440.

Eyelid Myoclonia with Absences, edited by J.S. Duncan and C.P. Panayiotopoulos
© 1996 John Libbey & Company Ltd, pp. 33–37.

Chapter 5

Eyelid myoclonia with absences in children: the Oxford experience

Z. Zaiwalla

Dr Zenobia Zaiwalla, Park Hospital for Children, Special Centre for Children with Epilepsy, Old Road, Headington, Oxford, OX3 7LQ

Seizures and seizure discharges related to eye closure have interested epileptologists for many years, starting with Gastaut & Tassinari's report in 1966 of two cases described as an 'exceptional type of visual reflex epilepsy'. Green (1968) described four cases (three were photosensitive) in whom closing the eyes triggered seizure activity. In three of the four cases the discharge continued until the eyes were shut. Light was not essential for the provocation of seizure activity, though a darkened room resulted in less intense seizure discharge. Green felt that the mechanism of seizure discharge on eye closure involved more than the physical factors of visual stimulation.

Darby *et al.* (1980) reported seven photosensitive patients who induced attacks by producing epileptiform paroxysms with slow eye closure, followed by sustained upward deviation of the eyes, the eye movement producing a characteristic oculographic artefact. They emphasized the importance of monitoring the oculogram during EEG studies.

More recently Barclay *et al.* (1993) reviewing the literature, identified two distinct forms of seizure induced by eyes-closed: those provoked by the absence of central vision (fixation-off seizures) and those related to actual movement of the eyelids. They also reported a woman in whom both mechanisms contributed to seizures induced by eyes-closed.

Brief seizure discharge on eye closure only, associated with photosensitivity and absences with eyelid myoclonia (EMA), was described by Jeavons in 1977 as a form of photosensitive epilepsy. Appleton *et al.* (1993) proposed that it should be recognised as a distinct epilepsy syndrome, starting around 3–7 years of age.

Case material

The Park Hospital for Children is a special centre for children with epilepsy, with a national referral base. In addition, the regional paediatric EEG service is provided from the Park Hospital covering Oxfordshire (population 590,400), Buckinghamshire (population 659,800) and Berkshire (population 767,800) and carries out about 2000 studies a year.

Children resistant to initial treatment have further studies with splitscreen/video EEG studies with or without simultaneous neuropsychological assessment or ambulatory cassette EEG recordings, to clarify the epilepsy syndrome further.

From an initial group of about 50 patients with drug resistant absence-like attacks, three patients with EMA were identified, using the diagnostic criteria suggested by Appleton *et al.* (1993). These cases will be compared with a case which appeared superficially similar, but with self induced attacks, followed by two other cases with sustained seizure discharges on eye closure.

Case studies

Group I Eyelid myoclonia with absences

Case 1

A 5 year old boy with developmental delay and hypotonia presented with recent onset of brief episodes of 'inaccessibility' with vertical eye movements and no other seizure type. No cause for the developmental delay was found on detailed neurometabolic investigations and neuroimaging. The family history was negative for epilepsy.

The standard EEG showed occasional spike discharges over both parieto-occipital areas, sometimes becoming more diffuse. Attempts at eye closure on request were unsuccessful, but there was a suggestion that the more diffuse epileptiform discharge occurred with spontaneous eye closure. Three episodes of EMA with absences associated with bursts of regular 3 Hz spike-wave discharge, lasting up to 3 s, occurred during the recording. In addition, he was photosensitive, with EMA occurring at some photic frequencies. The photoconvulsive response attenuated when one eye was covered.

Case 2

A 13 year old boy presented, with absences for many years, resistant to medication. The referring paediatric neurologist had noted that his father 'possibly had the same condition'.

A standard EEG at age 10 showed frequent 1–1.5 s paroxysms of generalized spike wave discharge on eye closure, and photic stimulation. At age 13 years he had 2 days of cassette EEG recording which included a period of splitscreen video EEG study with oculogram. The video EEG study confirmed that he was having EMA with no features suggestive of myoclonic absences. The paroxysms were not self induced and were not associated with significant interruption of cognitive function. The spike-wave paroxysms showed a diurnal pattern, occurring 30 to 40 times per hour in the first part of the day, decreasing to 7 to 10 per hour by late evening. Most of the paroxysms were associated with EMA. Covering one eye and dark glasses reduced the frequency of the epileptiform paroxysms to less than half. The spike-wave paroxysms, though present, were less frequent in sleep.

This boy is now maintained on a moderate dose of valproate to protect him from tonic clonic convulsions, and has been advised to use tinted glasses when socially acceptable.

Case 3

Case 3 is now 16 years old. She had two brief afebrile generalized tonic-clonic seizures at 18 months of age. A standard EEG at 3 years showed her to be photosensitive. At 9 years she was recognised to have frequent absence like attacks with eyes rolling up. A repeat standard EEG showed brief bursts of generalized spike wave discharge on eye closure, occurring less frequently with eyes open. The spike-wave discharge increased on hyperventilation and photic stimulation.

Her birth and developmental history was normal, but she is educationally 2 years behind her chronological age. She developed an eating disorder around 14 years of age.

The absence attacks remained resistant to treatment, increasing during periods of stress. A video

EEG study confirmed that she was having EMA which were not self induced, though increasing when under emotional pressure.

The parents have opted to discontinue antiepileptic drugs.

Group II Self induced seizures with photosensitivity

Case 4

This boy was referred at age 9 with a history of challenging behaviour and frequent "eye rolling" episodes since 5 years of age. The eye rolling episodes increased when tired or bored and had not responded to antiepileptic drugs. He also had occasional generalized tonic-clonic seizures.

A standard EEG at age 9 when on a combination of clobazam, ethosuximide and carbamazepine showed brief generalized irregular spike-wave discharges in the resting record with eyes open, not enhanced by eye closure. In addition, he was photosensitive.

During a splitscreen/video EEG study with recording of eye movements, he had frequent absence-like attacks, clinically resembling EMA, sometimes occurring in a cluster. However, the brief generalized spike-wave discharges which accompanied the eye movements were preceded by a slow eye movement, suggesting that the attacks were self induced. The epileptiform paroxysms could not be suppressed by wearing dark glasses or covering one eye. The discharge was infrequent in sleep.

He responded well to a combination of change in medication to valproate monotherapy, and psychotherapy.

Group III Seizure discharge persisting while eyes remain shut

Case 5

This boy was referred at 14 years of age. His epilepsy started at 18 months of age with a couple of floppy episodes. At 10 years he started having absence-like attacks and episodes with eye deviation to the right sometimes associated with falls. The attacks remain resistant to antiepileptic drugs. Two MRI scans and an FDG PET scan have been normal.

The standard EEG showed a left posterior temporal slow wave disturbance. In addition, as soon as he shut his eyes a continuous spike-wave discharge occurred bilaterally synchronously over both parieto-occipital and posterior temporal regions, more prominent on the left. With sustained eye closure the posterior discharge intermittently generalized. The discharge was suppressed by eye opening and did not increase on photic stimulation. A diagnosis of idiopathic occipital epilepsy was made.

A splitscreen/video EEG study with simultaneous neuropsychological assessment recording confirmed the response of the epileptiform discharge to eye closure in wakefulness. In addition, it was noted that the epileptiform activity generalized and became continuous in sleep. Episodes of recurrent head nodding with eye flickering and an episode of eye deviation to the right with the child appearing frightened showed ictal onset over the left posterior quadrant.

Neuropsychological testing during the EEG study at age 14 showed average ability with a verbal scale IQ score of 98 and performance scale IQ of 99 on the WISCIII. There was no significant difference in his performance with eyes open or shut. The overt seizures were infrequent and he seemed to be coping with his school work. However, 12 months later when he failed examinations the neuropsychological tests were repeated with splitscreen/video EEG recordings. The epileptiform activity had increased with occasional generalized spike-wave discharge with eyes open as well. Though no transient cognitive impairment could be demonstrated, he showed a fall in the verbal scale IQ score by 11 points (V = 87, P = 99), which reflected his difficulty in retrieving long term information and speed of processing information.

Clonazepam failed to suppress the continuous seizure activity in sleep or the discharges in wakefulness. There has been some reduction of overt seizures on a combination of vigabatrin and lamotrigine with tapering of carbamazepine.

Case 6

This 12 year old boy was referred to our EEG service with a recent single generalized tonic-clonic seizure. The standard EEG showed that as soon as he shut his eyes, brief paroxysms of generalized irregular spike-wave discharge occurred, which recurred every 2–3 s as long as the eyes remained shut. These paroxysms were associated with low amplitude eyelid flickering. The discharge attenuated on eye opening. It was difficult to be certain about photosensitivity as the paroxysms that coincided with photic stimulation may have been triggered by eye closure. A diagnosis of idiopathic generalized epilepsy was made.

A splitscreen/video EEG recording was carried out with neuropsychological assessment, including continuous tasks, repeated with eyes open and shut. This longer recording showed very infrequent generalized spike-wave paroxysms in wakefulness with eyes open. Recurrent brief paroxysms occurred with eyes shut, increasing in drowsiness, but decreasing in deeper stages of sleep. The neuropsychological assessment showed that though functioning in the average range, he had difficulty verbally generating items from categories with his eyes shut, and he commented that verbal response to auditory information was more difficult with eyes shut.

The parents opted not to start him on antiepileptic drugs, and 12 months on he has had no further generalized tonic-clonic seizures.

Conclusions

The review of our material confirms that EMA is a distinct but uncommon epilepsy syndrome, associated with photosensitivity in children. The seizures are often resistant to treatment. There is an overlap clinically and electrographically with children who are photosensitive and are able to self induce attacks with slow eye movements (Case 4). Stress may increase attacks in both conditions. Video EEG studies with recording of eye movements are necessary to differentiate the two seizure types.

EMA also has to be differentiated from epilepsy syndromes with sustained spike-wave discharge as long as eyes remain shut, as can occur in idiopathic occipital epilepsy (Case 5), and also in IGE syndromes with photosensitivity (Case 6). The discharge on eye closure in EMA decreases in darkness and reduces in sleep. Sustained discharge with eyes shut may increase in sleep, progressing to continuous spike-wave in slow wave sleep (CSWS) as in our Case 5.

EMA is not associated with significant interruption of cognitive function and there is no evidence of progressive cognitive deterioration with continuing seizures. A trial of broad spectrum antiepileptic drugs is certainly indicated, but if the seizures are resistant to treatment, it would be reasonable to maintain these children on a moderate dose of a single anticonvulsant only, to protect them against generalized tonic clonic convulsions seizures. This is not the case when sustained discharge occurs on eye closure. As shown by our Cases 5 and 6, the prolonged discharge does appear to interrupt cognitive function and especially if it is continuous in sleep may be associated with overall cognitive deterioration with time.

Detail video/EEG studies, including recording during sleep, and recording of eye movements, should be considered in all children with absence-like attacks resistant to first line antiepileptic drugs. This will enable recognition of the syndrome of EMA and other absence syndromes like myoclonic absences which are also drug resistant. In addition, simultaneous neuropsychological assessment may provide guidelines to when aggressive medical management is justified and when this is not indicated.

References

Appleton, R.E., Panayiotopoulos, C.P., Acombe, B.A., Beirne, M. (1993): Eyelid myoclonia with typical absences: an epilepsy syndrome. *J. Neurol. Neurosurg. Psychiatry* **56,** 1312–1316.

Barclay, C.L., Murphy, W.F., Lee, M.A., Darwish, Z.H. (1993): Unusual form of seizures induced by eye closure. *Epilepsia* **34,** 289–293.

Darby, C.E., de Korte, R.A., Binnie, C.D., Wilkins, A.J. (1980): The self induction of epileptic seizures by eye closure. *Epilepsia* **21,** 31–42.

Gastaut, H., Tassinari, C.A. (1966): Triggering mechanisms in epilepsy. *Epilepsia* **7,** 85–138.

Green, J.B. (1968): Seizures on closing the eyes. Electro encephalographic studies. *Neurology* **18,** 391–396.

Jeavons, P.M. (1977): Nosological problems of myoclonic epilepsies in childhood and adolescence. *Dev. Med. Child Neurol.* **19,** 3–8.

Eyelid Myoclonia with Absences, edited by J.S. Duncan and C.P. Panayiotopoulos
© 1996 John Libbey & Company Ltd, pp. 39–48.

Chapter 6

The spectrum of childhood epilepsies with eyelid myoclonia

C.D. Ferrie, [1]A. Agathonikou, [1]A. Parker, R.O. Robinson and [1]C.P. Panayiotopoulos

Deptartment of Paediatric Neurology, Guy's Hospital, London; [1]Deptartment of Clinical Neurophysiology & Epilepsies, St Thomas' Hospital, London

Movements of the eyelids are common ictal symptoms in children with various epilepsy syndromes. There has been little attempt to systematically define such phenomena or to study their significance. In general, the movements usually appear relatively trivial, described as 'flickering' or 'fluttering', and are considered of little or no significance either to classification or in predicting prognosis. The exception to this is eyelid myoclonia, identified as a hallmark of eyelid myoclonia with absences (EMA), a myoclonic epilepsy syndrome classified amongst the idiopathic generalized epilepsies (Jeavons, 1977) and often presenting a highly distinctive clinical picture with a prognosis quite different from many other childhood IGE (Panayiotopoulos, 1994; 1996). However, ictal eyelid myoclonia is not confined to EMA. In this chapter we compare eyelid myoclonia occurring in children with EMA to that seen in other epilepsies.

An immediate problem is to determine what constitutes eyelid myoclonia as distinct from other eyelid movements. Some doubt whether such a distinction exists (Hirsch & Marescaux, 1995). Most parents who describe the phenomena in their children emphasize the violence of the eyelid movements. However, reliance on eye witness accounts is unreliable as others use less evocative language; the importance of video and video-EEG documentation therefore hardly needs stating. Following the definition of myoclonia as a rapid, involuntary muscle contraction (Niedermeyer, 1993), eyelid myoclonia is a sudden involuntary jerk of the eyelid which can be single or multiple, rhythmic or arrhythmic. Whilst often very pronounced, it may be subtle. Eyelid myoclonia has an involuntary, forced or compulsive quality unlike other ictal eyelid movements which usually resemble physiological eyelid blinking and are best viewed as automatisms and are release phenomena. Eyelid myoclonia, especially in EMA, is often accompanied by a tonic component in the involved muscles, tonic upward deviation of the eyes or more widespread myoclonia of the head, shoulders or whole body (Giannakodimos & Panayiotopoulos, 1996).

No epilepsy syndrome is defined by one ictal symptom; whilst eyelid myoclonia is a prerequisite for the diagnosis of EMA, not all patients with eyelid myoclonia, even when associated with

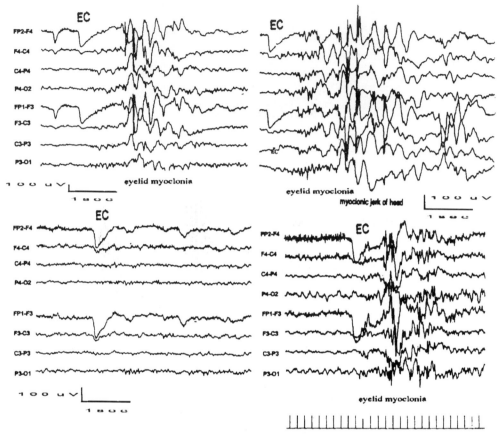

Fig 1. Video-EEG from Case 1 at 10 years of age. On eye closure brief bursts of generalized polyspikes and slow waves occurred with accompanying eyelid myoclonia, either with (top right) or without (top left) more widespread myoclonic phenomena. Not all eye closures were accompanied by such abnormalities (bottom left). Similar abnormalities on IPS (bottom right).

idiopathc generalized epilepsy and typical absence seizures, have EMA. It is the non-fortuitous clustering of various signs, symptoms, etc. which constitutes an epilepsy syndrome (Commission on Classification and Terminology, 1989). In EMA, the precipitating effect of eye closure, the associated brief and mild absences and photosensitivity are as important as eyelid myoclonia in defining the syndrome.

Eyelid myoclonia in children with idiopathic generalized epilepsies

Minor eyelid phenomena during typical absence seizures are relatively common in children with childhood and juvenile absence epilepsies (Aicardi, 1994); parents often report eyelid 'flickering' or 'fluttering'. On video-EEG this is usually revealed as blinking movements, similar to physiological blinking, either randomly or at around 3 Hz. Whether mild eyelid myoclonia occurs in these epilepsies has not yet been firmly established. Dalla Bernardina *et al.*, (1989) reported eyelid myoclonia as a symptom in benign myoclonic epilepsy of infancy, 'petit-mal absences', 'petit-mal + grand mal epilepsy' and juvenile myoclonic epilepsy. However, as testified by the terminology,

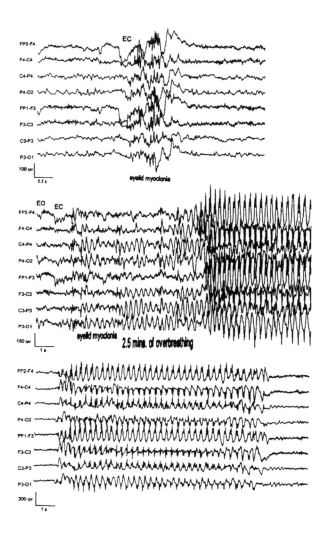

Fig 2. Video-EEG recorded from case 3 at 10 years of age.
Top: Generalized polyspike and wave discharges associated with eyelid myoclonia on eye closure.
Middle: Similar discharge on eye closure accompanied by eyelid myoclonia but followed by typical absence lasting more than 8 s and accompanied by severe impairment of consciousness and simple automatisms.
Bottom: Spontaneous typical absence seizure without eyelid myoclonia.

the syndrome classification were less rigorous than is the current standard and although polygraphic recordings were made, video-EEG was not.

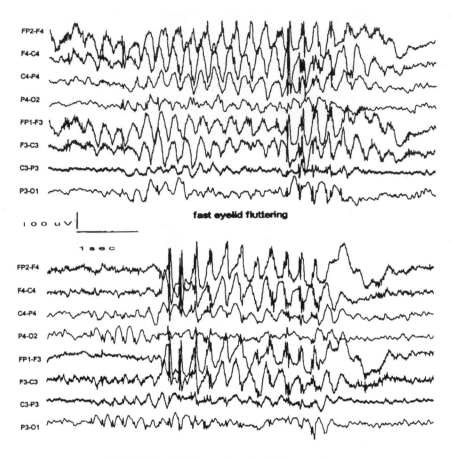

Fig 3. Video-EEG from Case 8 at 11 years of age
Top: spontaneous discharge with accompanying eyelid myoclonia. Eye closure
abnormalities were not seen.
Bottom: Similar discharge during overbreathing with breath-counting. No eyelid
myoclonia occurred during the ictus but the patient repeated the number '5'.

Eyelid myoclonia with absences: typical cases

Giannakodimos & Panayiotopoulos in this volume (chapter 8) and previously (1996) have proposed a definition of EMA which is significantly stricter than that employed previously. In particular, other authors have permitted the occurrence of typical absence seizures independently of those with eyelid myoclonia (Appleton *et al.*, 1993; Appleton, 1995). We have identified three children in the last 2 years, two of whom are presented below, who fulfil the stricter definition. An example is :

Case 1

A 10 year old girl with a normal perinatal and general medical history with onset of seizures around the age of 4 years. Seizures were brief, consisting of tonic upward deviation of the eyes with marked eyelid myoclonia. More severe seizures were accompanied by a retropulsive jerk of her head, shoulders and sometimes limbs, on occasions leading to falls and a diagnosis of 'drop attacks'. All seizures were brief and accompanied by, at most, a mild impairment of consciousness. The vast majority were light-induced, with sudden increases in background illumination, especially going into bright sunshine, being powerful provocation. Watching TV or playing video-games were less powerful stimuli. Occasional independent myoclonic jerks of her limbs were described. Typical absences unaccompanied by eyelid phenomena have not occurred; neither as yet, have generalized tonic-clonic seizures. Treatment with sodium valproate was unsuccessful. Vigabatrin was of no benefit and carbamazepine exacerbated seizures and led to occasional episodes of urinary incontinence. Sodium valproate combined both with ethosuximide and with lamotrigine greatly reduced but did not eliminate seizures. There was a strong family history of photosensitive seizures. (see this volume, chapter 13). On video-EEG frequent seizures with eyelid myoclonia occurred mainly on eye closure (Fig. 1).

We have not systematically investigated the contentious issue of self induction of seizures in children with EMA (Darby *et al.* 1980). Behaviours such as compulsive close-up TV viewing, hand waving ('sunflower manoeuvre'), and horizontal head nodding observed on a family video-recording, indicate probable self-induction of a minority of seizures in this patient. However, her parents were certain that the majority of seizures were not self-induced. On viewing home video-recordings of children, it is apparent that seizures with eyelid myoclonia occur during relatively complex tasks, including catching balls and caring for pets.

Case 2

Now aged 17 years, he had an unremarkable past history. From the age of 8 years he had frequent episodes with tonic upward deviation of his eyes and eyelid 'flickering' without interruption of activity. A vivid description was given of him dashing for the tape in a race with, "His eyes flickering almost continuously." Seizures were provoked by sudden exposure to sunlight, social embarrassment or else apparently spontaneously. Treatment with carbamazepine was unsuccessful but sodium valproate partially controlled seizures. There was no family history of note. Standard EEG consistently showed generalized spike and wave discharges with photosensitivity. Two video-EEGs were performed. These revealed characteristic EEG features of EMA, including brief generalized spike, multiple spike and wave discharges on eye closure accompanied by fast eyelid flicker.

Previous studies have demonstrated that in adults with EMA, particularly those on correct treatment, video-EEG may reveal the characteristic eye closure EEG abnormalities accompanied by fast eyelid flicker, rather than the more violent myoclonia witnessed clinically and recorded on video or previous video-EEGs (Giannakodimos & Panayiotopoulos, 1996). Despite the smaller amplitude of such movements, they share the other features of eyelid myoclonia and are probably a minor manifestation of it. We conclude that the diagnosis of EMA is appropriate when other features are typical. These milder eyelid abnormalities may reflect natural variation in severity seen in all epilepsy syndromes, reduction in severity occurring with increasing age or appropriate medication.

EMA appears to be a life-long condition and the definition given previously emphasizes its evolutionary nature. In paediatric practice only the early stages are seen which probably accounts for the fact that none of our cases had generalized tonic-clonic seizures; correct diagnosis and appropriate management may prevent their occurrence. Similarly, in childhood cases we have not seen eyelid myoclonia unaccompanied by EEG changes as reported in adults (Giannakodimos & Panayiotopoulos, 1996).

Eyelid myoclonia in other idiopathic epilepsies, including possible atypical cases of EMA

We have seen a number of children with idiopathic generalized epilepsies who have some but not all of the key features required for a diagnosis of EMA. Examples of these are presented below in order to illustrate the spectrum in which the symptom of eyelid myoclonia occurs and to stimulate further studies in this area.

Case 3

Now aged 9 years with an unremarkable past history, she had onset of seizures at 6 years of age. These consisted of episodes lasting up to 45 seconds of psychomotor arrest, accompanied by head slumping, either to the right or to the left. Her parents did not describe eyelid phenomena during such episodes. However, on some occasions her attacks were associated with falls, suggesting a myoclonic component, and mild eyelid myoclonia was observed on several occasions in the clinic. The maximum seizure frequency was 2–3/day. There was no family history of note. Sodium valproate reduced but did not eliminate her seizures. Two video-EEGs both showed characteristic eye-closure related abnormalities accompanied by prominent eyelid myoclonia. However, in addition she had typical absences, both preceded by and independently of seizures with eyelid myoclonia (Fig. 2). According to the previously cited definition, independent absences, prolonged absences and absences with severe impairment of consciousness are against EMA as a diagnosis. On the other hand the prominent myoclonic component to her seizures, the marked photosensitivity and the eye-closure related EEG abnormalities are incompatible with childhood or juvenile absence epilepsies (Panayiotopoulos, 1994, 1996). The definition of EMA was based on a study in adults; in children the clinical spectrum may be wider.

Case 4

Now aged 7 years, she presented to the ophthalmologists with a diagnosis of very frequent 'occulogyric crises' starting at 5 years of age. These consisted of tonic upward deviation of the eyes with 'eyelid blinking', accompanied by brief psychomotor arrest. The attacks were more common in bright sunlight, pleasurable but, according to the patient, not self-induced despite descriptions of compulsive close-up TV viewing. Although neurologically normal, she struggles to keep up in class and has behavioural problems. Sodium valproate alone or combined with lamotrigine failed. EMA was suspected clinically and video-EEG revealed her to be highly photosensitive, with myoclonic head jerks and fast eyelid blinking/eyelid myoclonia during ictal discharges. Despite this no eye closure related abnormalities were seen in the remainder of the EEG. She has a sister who has had two generalized tonic-clonic convulsions, one whilst watching TV. In children on appropriate treatment with clinical features compatible with EMA, the lack of EEG confirmation of the typical clinical and EEG eye closure related abnormalities does not exclude the diagnosis of EMA. However, we consider these to be so fundamental that the diagnosis is in doubt until they are demonstrated. This is especially the case in those in whom habitual seizures, not related to eye closure, are recorded.

Case 5

This girl with an unremarkable past and family history presented at 12 years of age with four seizures occurring over the previous 34 years. All were characterized by sudden loss of consciousness and hypotonia causing her to fall. Seizures lasted up to 2 minutes and no other ictal features were described. Three seizures occurred whilst the TV was on, although she denies watching it at the time, and the other whilst working on a VDU screen. There was no history suggestive of other seizures. Standard and video-EEG revealed photosensitivity and eye closure induced brief generalized bursts of spike, multiple spike and wave accompanied by inconstant eyelid myoclonia/fast fluttering. Treatment was refused.

Case 6

This boy presented at 12 years of age having had six seizures in the previous 6 months. The first two occurred whilst watching TV, the others apparently spontaneously. Each began with visual symptoms, including complete or left hemi-field blindness, 'flickering' of the visual field or apparent hallucinations causing him to cry out, "Get him off me." After a variable time up to 15 minutes impairment of consciousness and secondary generalisation sometimes occurred. His mother had two seizures, one whilst watching TV, as a teenager. Standard and video-EEGs have revealed him to be highly photosensitive with frequent short, posteriorly predominant, bursts of high voltage polyspike and wave discharges, either bilaterally or independently right or left. Eye-closure provoked discharges whose morphology was identical to that seen in EMA; despite this no eyelid myoclonia phenomena were seen. Poor follow-up precludes comment on response to treatment.

The latter two cases clearly do not have EMA. Indeed the symptomatology of case 6 suggests partial onset of seizures. However, both had video-EEG findings which raised the possibility of EMA. They illustrate the importance of not attaching undue weight to any single electro-clinical finding.

EMA is, in general, among the most distinctive of the idiopathic generalized epilepsies. The existence of patients who may have EMA but are atypical and of patients who do not have EMA, but share with it common features, should not be used as an argument against its existence but should be a stimulus to further research. Meanwhile, the dangers of 'forcing' atypical cases into existing syndromes, particularly in research studies, has been stressed (Panayiotopoulos, 1995).

Cryptogenic/symptomatic epilepsies

Eyelid phenomena are commonly seen during non-convulsive seizures in children with cryptogenic and symptomatic generalized epilepsies. These include eyelid blinking and flutter. True eyelid myoclonia is less common but certainly occurs, especially in children with generalized epilepsies, and appears to have been reported previously as EMA (De Marco, 1989). Some authors report 'rapid forced eye blinking' at seizure onset in occipital lobe partial seizures (Kotagal, 1993). The following three cases illustrate the occurrence of the symptom of eyelid myoclonia in symptomatic/cryptogenic epilepsies.

Case 7

This woman (reported previously, Ferrie *et al.*, 1995, case 7), now aged 22 years, had a family history of 'epilepsy'. Following some neonatal respiratory problems, she was well until the onset of absences at 3 years of age, with generalized tonic-clonic seizures, including episodes of convulsive status, starting soon after. She was moderately retarded, of short stature and developed hypothyroidism as a young adult. Through most of her life she has had absences at a pyknolepsy-like frequency. These were of variable duration, usually with moderate or mild impairment of consciousness. During them adversive head movements to the right were frequent, along with prominent 'jerking' of the eyelids. Although MRI was normal, significant hypometabolism of the right temporal lobe was revealed by inter-ictal[18] flurodeoxyglucose positron emission tomography. During video-EEG frequent, mainly short absences were recorded. These were often, but not always, associated with eyelid myoclonia. The patient was photosensitive. Seizures mostly occurred with eyes closed and eye-closure related abnormalities were not seen.

Case 8

This 11 year old boy had the onset in infancy of a mixed seizure disorder with segmental and massive myoclonias, atypical absences and aggressive outbursts, probably ictal in origin. He is globally delayed (IQ: 50–55), with significant behavioural problems. Many of his absences manifest with psychomotor arrest and head drops; at other times there is tonic upward eye deviation with 'eyelid myoclonia or blinking'. Treatment with various agents, including sodium valproate, has failed to control his seizures. His sister, who also has learning difficulties has a similar form of epilepsy, but due to family disruption further details are not known. Previous EEG examinations revealed excess slow activity accompanied by bursts and runs of multiple spike and wave at frequencies varying from 2.5–4 Hz. Intermittent photic stimulation evoked generalized photocon-

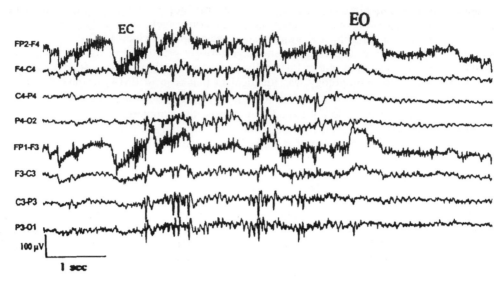

Fig 4. Video-EEG from case 9 at 16 years of age.
These eyes-closed discharges were inconstantly associated with eyelid myoclonia.

vulsive responses. Variable focal features were evident. Video-EEG at 11 years of age showed excess background slow with frequent bursts of high amplitude multiple spike and wave, with at times a marked right frontal emphasis. These were accompanied by impairment of consciousness, backward head jerks, tonic eye deviation, mainly to the left, and variable eyelid myoclonia, at times marked. Hyperventilation greatly increased these abnormalities.

Investigations have revealed no cause for this patient's seizures and he has been classified as having cryptogenic generalized epilepsy.

Case 9

This man, now 19 years old and of Colombian origin, was globally delayed (WISC score = 68) and had a chromosomal anomaly consisting of two cell lines – one normal 46, XY, the other with 47 chromosomes including a ring chromosome of E group size. From the age of 6–8 months he had shown frequent eyelid myoclonia, latterly provoked by TV and video-games. At 4 and 7 years of age, following withdrawal of medication, he had generalized tonic-clonic seizures and at 7 years of age also had a number of drop attacks, the exact nature of which is not clear. Gelastic seizures occurred between 17 and 18 years of age. Clinical absences were never described although EEG at 9 years of age showed generalized spike, multiple spike and slow wave discharges and generalized photoconvulsive response on intermittent photic stimulation. Eyelid myoclonia has continued despite medication which has included sodium valproate and clobazam. Video-EEG at 16 years of age showed frequent fast occipital spikes bilaterally with alternating side emphasis with eyes closed, sometimes accompanied by eyelid myoclonia (Fig 4). At 17 years of age similar spikes were provoked by binocular and monocular intermittent photic stimulation. MRI and [18]flurodeoxyglucose PET scans were normal.

Diagnostic confusion between patients with symptomatic or cryptogenic epilepsies who show ictal eyelid myoclonia and those with the syndrome of EMA will rarely be a problem if the clinical background is considered in detail, mental retardation, neurological signs, etc. being incompatible with an idiopathic epilepsy. Similarly, although some excess slow activity may be seen in poorly controlled idiopathic epilepsies and those on antiepileptic drugs, a marked excess suggest a cryptogenic/symptomatic aetiology of seizures. Focal EEG abnormalities are common in EMA but when severe or persistent are likely to indicate an underlying structural abnormality. Seizures in EMA are brief and stereotyped; occasional independent myoclonic jerks of the limbs/body and generalized tonic-clonic seizures are the only other seizure types which occur (Giannakodimos & Panayiotopoulos, 1996). In cryptogenic/symptomatic cases eyelid myoclonia is an inconstant ictal feature, and may be associated with seizures both of variable duration and of different types (for example, atypical absences and partial seizures). Tonic, atonic and partial seizures are incompatible with the diagnosis of EMA. Finally, we have not seen activation of seizures by eye closure in symptomatic/cryptogenic cases.

Conclusions

For anyone who has witnessed eyelid myoclonia, either in real-time or on video, it is seldom difficult to differentiate it from non-myoclonic phenomena. It is important to stress, however, that its mere identification is insufficient to diagnose the syndrome of EMA. With appropriate investigations, particularly the use of video-EEG, differentiation of EMA from cryptogenic/symptomatic epilepsies is rarely a problem. Whether the occurrence of eyelid myoclonia in such epilepsies is of diagnostic or prognostic significance has not been investigated. However, they may eventually provide clues by which the aetiopathogenesis of the phenomena is elucidated. The precise boundaries of the syndrome of EMA and other idiopathic generalized epilepsies with eyelid myoclonia are still controversial. Currently inclusion of only the most typical cases is more likely to advance understanding, particularly of the molecular genetics, of the condition, hopefully avoiding some of the problems seen with juvenile myoclonic epilepsy (Gardiner, 1995). Not withstanding this, the phenotypic expression of EMA may be wider than is generally recognized now.

Acknowledgment

We thank the Special Trustees of St. Thomas' Hospital for the financial support of our studies in the syndromic diagnosis of epilepsies.

References

Aicardi, J. (1994): *Epilepsy in children,* 2nd edn., New York: Raven Press.

Appleton, R.E. (1995): Eyelid myoclonia with absences. In: *Typical absences and related epileptic syndromes,* eds. J.S. Duncan & C.P. Panayiotopoulos, pp. 213–220. Edinburgh: Churchill Livingstone.

Appleton, R.E., Panayiotopoulos, C.P., Acomb, B.A. & Beirne, M. (1993): Eyelid myoclonia with typical absences: an epilepsy syndrome. *J. Neurol. Neurosurg. Psychiatry* **56,** 1312–1316.

Commission on Classification and Terminology of the International League Against Epilepsy (1989): Proposal for revised clinical and electroencephalographic classification of epilepsies and epileptic syndromes. *Epilepsia* **30,** 389–399.

Dalla Bernardina, B., Sgro, V. & Fontanna, E., *et al.*. (1989): Eyelid myoclonia with absences. In: *Reflex seizures and reflex epilepsies.* eds. A. Beaumanoir, H. Gastaut, R. Naquet, pp. 193–200. Geneva: Medicine & Hygiene.

Darby, C.E., de Korte, R.A., Binnie, C.D. & Wilkins, A.J. (1980): The self-induction of epileptic seizures by eye closure. *Epilepsia* **21,** 31–42.

De Marco, P. (1989): Eyelid myoclonia with absences (EMA) in two monovular twins. *Clin. Electroencephalogr.* **20,** 193–195.

Ferrie, C.D., Giannakodimos, S., Robinson, R.O. & Panayiotopoulos, C.P. (1995): Symptomatic typical absence seizures. In: *Typical absences and related epileptic syndromes,* eds. J.S. Duncan & C.P. Panayiotopoulos, pp. 241–252. London: Churchill Livingstone.

Gardiner, M. (1995): Genetics of human typical absence syndromes. In: *Typical absences and related epileptic syndromes.* eds. J.S. Duncan, C.P. Panayiotopoulos, pp. 320–327. London: Churchill Livingstone.

Giannakodimos, S. & Panayiotopoulos, C.P. (1996): Eyelid myoclonia with absences in adults: a clinical and video-EEG study. *Epilepsia* (in press).

Hirsch, E. & Marescaux, C. (1995): How should epileptic syndromes with typical absences be classified. In: *Typical absences and related epilepsy syndromes.* eds. J.S. Duncan & C.P. Panayiotopoulos, pp. 310–314. London: Churchill Livingstone.

Jeavons, P.M. (1977): Nosololgical problems of myoclonic epilepsies in childhood and adolescence. *Dev. Med. Child Neurol.* **19,** 38.

Kotagal, P. (1993): Psychomotor seizures: clinical and EEG findings. In: *The treatment of epilepsy: principles and practice,* ed. E. Wyllie, pp. 378–392. Philadelphia: Lee & Febiger.

Niedermeyer, E. (1993): Epileptic seizure disorders. In: *Electroencephalography: basic principles, clinical applications, and related fields,* 3rd edn., eds. E. Niedermeyer & F. Lopes Da Silva, pp. 461–564. Baltimore: Urban & Schwartzenberg.

Panayiotopoulos, C.P. (1994): The clinical spectrum of typical absence seizures and absence epilepsies. In: *Idiopathic generalized epilepsies,* eds. A. Malafosse, P. Genton, E. Hirsch, C. Marescaux, D. Broglin & R. Bernasconi, pp. 73–83. London: John Libbey.

Panayiotopoulos, C.P. (1995): Typical absences are syndrome related. In: *Typical absences and related epilepsy syndromes,* eds. J.S. Duncan & C.P. Panayiotopoulos, pp. 304–310. London: Churchill Livingstone.

Panayiotopoulos, C.P. (1996): Absence epilepsies: childhood, juvenile and myoclonic absence epilepsy, eyelid myoclonia with absences and other related epileptic syndromes with typical absence seizures. In: *Epilepsy: a comprehensive textbook (volume 3),* eds., J.E. Engel & T.A. Pedley. New York: Raven Press (in press).

Eyelid Myoclonia with Absences, edited by J.S. Duncan and C.P. Panayiotopoulos
© 1996 John Libbey & Company Ltd, pp. 49–56.

Chapter 7

Eyelid myoclonia with absences in adults: comparison with other absence seizures

S.J.M. Smith

The National Hospital for Neurology and Neurosurgery, Queen Square, London, WC1N 3BG, UK

Eyelid myoclonia with typical absences (EMA) is considered to be an idiopathic generalized epilepsy syndrome, comprising a number of distinct clinical features (Appleton *et al.* 1993). Typically, brief absences are accompanied by eyelid myoclonia, with retropulsion of the eyeballs and occasionally the head. Seizures begin in childhood and precipitation by sunlight is often a characteristic feature in the early history. The electroencephalogram (EEG) shows generalized high amplitude spikes or polyspike and wave during seizures, with photosensitivity. However, although there appear to be distinct electroclinical features, eyelid myoclonia with typical absences has not yet been recognized as a separate syndrome by the International League against Epilepsy.

The prevalence of this syndrome is unknown. The number of reported cases is small, and even in specialist centres with a particular interest in the condition, it appears to be very uncommon (Appleton *et al.* 1993). It is not clear whether this represents true rarity or underdiagnosis. The ease with which the clinical features of the seizures of EMA can be distinguished from other types of absences is uncertain. Particular difficulties may arise in recognizing the brevity of the absence compared with the longer duration of impaired consciousness in childhood absence epilepsy, and the contrast between the myoclonic eyelid movements of EMA and the eyelid fluttering or flickering in other absences. It is usual in EMA for seizures to perisist into adulthood, but it is unclear whether the clinical characteristics of the absences remain the same as in children, or evolve with age.

To determine whether there are distinctive clinical features which permit a diagnosis of EMA in adults, a series of patients with absences and rapid eyelid movements has been evaluated. Cases were drawn from a large population of adult patients with epilepsy attending the National Hospital for Neurology and Neurosurgery and the Chalfont Centre for Epilepsy.

Patients and methods

Eleven patients were identified between 1993 and 1995 who fulfilled the criterion of absences associated with rapid eyelid movements. All cases were studied with video telemetry to document seizures. In two patients, there were no attacks during the period of video EEG study, and clinical features were assessed by a careful history with witness accounts.

Eyelid myoclonia with absences

There were five patients whose seizures were considered to show the characteristics of eyelid myoclonia with absences (Table 1).

Case 1

Case 1 was a 23 year old female. Seizures began in late childhood with absences and eyelid myoclonia, often occurring when she went out into bright sunlight. Generalized tonic-clonic seizures were rare. There was no history of myoclonic jerks. There was a family history of epilepsy: an uncle had generalized tonic-clonic seizure and her brother had had two seizures whilst using a computer. Seizures were documented in the patient during hyperventilation and photic stimulation, and consisted of brief episodes of rapid eyelid movements, with uprolling of her eyes during photic stimulation. The EEG accompaniment was rhythmic generalized slow activity but no definite spikes (Fig. 1). Dramatic improvement in seizure control was achieved with a combination of sodium valproate and ethosuximide.

Case 2

This 22 year old male had onset of frequent absences with eyelid and head movements at the age of 9 years. He had occasional generalized tonic-clonic seizures; early morning myoclonic jerks developed during his teenage years. Family history was negative. An EEG at the age of 9 years showed polyspike and slow wave discharges and photosensitivity. MRI was normal. Very frequent seizures were documented during telemetry. The attacks were brief (2–3 s) with retropulsion of the eyeballs and rapid eyelid movements. The high frequency of seizures was thought to contribute to impaired functioning on psychometric testing; there was, however, no definite history of status.

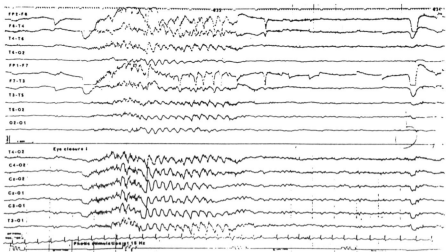

Fig. 1. Case 1 of the EMA group. Electrographic accompaniments of absence seizure elicited by eye closure during photic stimulation at 15 Hz. A high frequency discharge occurs with the eyelid myoclonia, followed by rhythmical slow activity but no clear spikes.

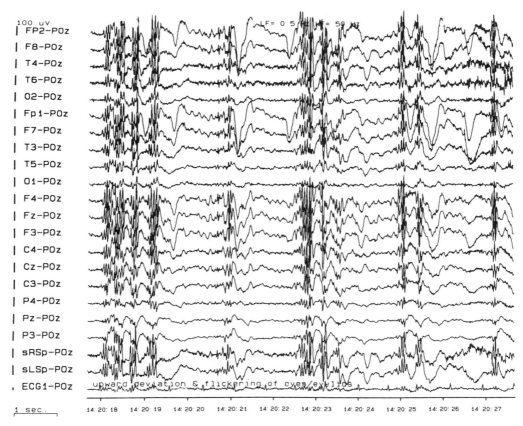

100 uv

| FP2-POz
| F8-POz
| T4-POz
| T6-POz
| 02-POz
| Fp1-POz
| F7-POz
| T3-POz
| T5-POz
| 01-POz
| F4-POz
| Fz-POz
| F3-POz
| C4-POz
| Cz-POz
| C3-POz
| P4-POz
| Pz-POz
| P3-POz
| sRSp-POz
| sLSp-POz
, ECG1-POz

LF= 0 5 HF = 50 Hz

upward deviation & flickering of eyes/eyelids

1 sec.

14 20:18   14 20:19   14 20:20   14 20:21   14 20:22   14 20:23   14 20:24   14 20:25   14 20:26   14 20:27

Fig. 2. Case 4 of the EMA group. EEG during episode of eyelid myoclonia and absence status. Frequent very brief seizures are associated with rapid polyspiking and subsequent spike and slow discharge.

Ethosuximide and sodium valporate had been tried separately with little effect, but a combination of ethosuximide and lamotrigine led to a rapid and substantial reduction in seizures.

Case 3

Case 3 was a 15 year old female, with absences and rapid eyelid flickering from the age of 8 years. At the time of seizure onset, her EEG showed generalized spike and wave and photosensitivity. There were no generalized tonic-clonic seizures or myoclonic jerks. A paternal half sister had seizures of unknown type. At the age of 11 years, the patient had an episode of absence status following treatment for lobar pneumonia. Since then she has had spontaneous episodes of continuous absence seizures lasting for 24 hours, with up to one episode per month. Seizures documented on telemetry showed brief absences with rapid eyelid movements and uprolling of eyes.

Case 4

Absences in this 27 year old female were first diagnosed at the age of 15 years. There was no history of seizures evoked by environmental photic stimuli, generalized tonic-clonic seizures or myoclonic jerks. Family history was negative. Previous EEGs had shown generalized spike or polyspike and wave discharges, but no photosensitivity. MRI was normal. The patient described seizures occurring in clusters, and being 'blank for 24 hours'. During the telemetry study, she had continuous brief

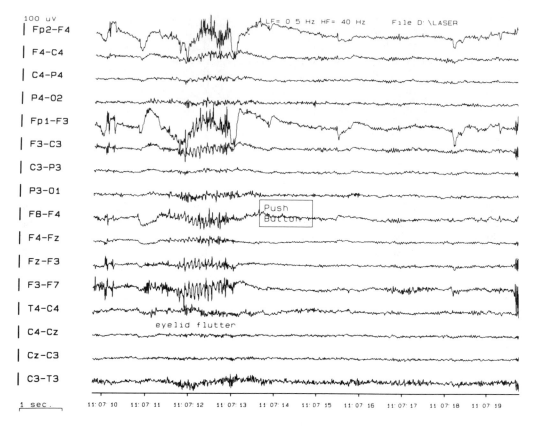

Fig. 3. Case 1 of the self inducing group. The EEG during rapid eyelid flutter and retropulsion of eyeballs show muscle artefact but no spike and wave discharge.

absences with retropulsion of eyes and very rapid myoclonic jerks of the eyelids over a 24 hour period (Fig. 2). Moderate seizure control was obtained with combined phenytoin and ethosuximide.

Case 5

This 41 year old man had absences and eyelid flickering from the age of 3 years. Infrequent generalized tonic-clonic seizures occurred in his teens; there was no history of myoclonic jerks. His father had blank spells as a youth and a paternal aunt had generalized convulsions. The seizures had become gradually more frequent, and at the time of assessment, he had many seizures per day, worse in the early morning. A witness account described a blank stare and rapid fluttering of the eyelids for a few seconds. On occasions, the seizures would become continuous with obtundation lasting for 36 hours. EEGs as a young adult had shown generalized spike and wave activity. MRI was normal. Monotherapy with sodium valproate led to a significant reduction in seizures.

Typical absences

Two patients had brief absences accompanied by eyelid flickering but no clear myoclonia or eyeball retropulsion. These cases were considered to have typical absence seizures as a manifestation of idiopathic generalized epilepsy.

Case 1

This 21 year old man had onset of absences at the age of 7 years, and occasional generalized tonic-clonic seizures. Family history was positive: a paternal aunt and her children had epilepsy. EEGs as a child had shown spike or polyspike and wave with photosensitivity. His current seizures consisted of frequent absences which were brief and associated with rapid flickering of the eyelids. Most of the absences were associated with generalized spike and wave activity, but some had no EEG accompaniment. Myoclonic jerks of the head and limbs occurred at other times, exacerbated by bright sunlight. Response to sodium valproate had been excellent in the past, but side effects limited its use. Moderate seizure control was achieved with combined phenytoin, ethosuximide and carbamazepine. MRI showed a small circumscribed white matter lesion in the left frontal lobe, thought to be of no relevance.

Case 2

Case 2 was a 38 year old woman, with seizures starting in early childhood. Initially, seizures were brief generalized tonic-clonic seizures; absences were not documented until several years later. Family history was positive, with seizures in her maternal grandmother. Early EEG data were not available. At the time of study, she had 2–5 s runs of generalized slow activity associated with ill defined spikes in the frontal regions on EEG. Some of these episodes were accompanied by eyelid flickering but no retropulsion of the eyeballs. The patient did not report these as absences. Photic stimulation caused distress and ill defined generalized sharp and slow activity was seen at 18 Hz.

Atypical absences

Two cases had absences that were considered to be atypical on the basis of the seizure pattern and associated clinical features.

Case 1

Case 1 was a 57 year old woman, born at 44 weeks and requiring resuscitation. Developmental delay was noted from 5 months, with subsequent quadriparesis and moderate mental retardation. Absences began at the age of 12 years, with jerking of the eyelids, uprolling of the eyes, clonic jerking of the arms and incontinence. There was no history of generalized tonic-clonic seizures. Family history was negative. Recorded seizures showed sudden dropping of the head, eyes deviated upwards and to the right, rapid eyelid movements and orofacial automatisms, of duration up to 1 minute. Rhythmic sharp and slow activity maximal in the parasagittal regions was seen on the ictal EEG.

Case 2

This was a 33 year old woman, who had been a full term delivery, with maternal eclampsia. Myoclonic absences had occurred from age 6 months, with moderate intellectual impairment. Generalized tonic-clonic seizures began at 12 years, with infrequent GTC status. At the time of study, generalized seizures were rare, but myoclonic absences were occurring at the rate of up to 20 per day. These consisted of absences, eyelid and perioral myoclonia, head nodding and brief jerks of her arms. Hyperventilation increased the frequency of attacks. The EEG accompaniments were generalized irregular 33.5 Hz spike or polyspike and wave discharges, with shifting lateralisation.

Non-epileptic or self induced attacks

Two patients appeared to have self induced attacks, in addition to other seizures.

Case 1

This was a 32 year old woman who had had a febrile convulsion at 12 months and persistent seizures from the age of 5 years. Seizures comprised generalized tonic-clonic convulsions and absences with eyelid fluttering and upper limb myoclonia. She had severe mental retardation. A sister also had epilepsy and retardation (their parents are second cousins). Telemetry identified very frequent episodes of eyelid flutter, during which she looked upwards. The EEG showed muscle artefact only (Fig. 3). There was no photosensitivity. A single absence was recorded; this consisted of a blank stare and less rapid eye blinking, with generalized spike and wave.

Case 2

This 30 year old woman had a 2 year history of seizures beginning after treatment for psychotic depression. She had occasional generalized tonic-clonic seizures and absences. Generalized spike and wave discharge was seen on the EEG; there was no photosensitivity. Recorded attacks consisted of eyes rolling upwards, rapid eye blinking but no definite impairment of consciousness, followed by a fall to ground, during which she lay still and unresponsive for several minutes. No EEG change was seen other than artefact.

Discussion

The attacks in the four groups of patients share common clinical features. The combination of eyelid myoclonia and retropulsion of eyeballs is characteristic of EMA, but upward movements of the eyes were also seen in the atypical absences and self inducers. However, there were other features in the latter two groups that allow distinction from EMA. In the atypical absences, there was additional myoclonus of the face and limbs, and both patients had evidence of underlying neurological disease and mental retardation. The self induced episodes could be distinguished by the absence of generalized spike wave discharge in the EEG. Furthermore, the cases with self induced attacks had either mental retardation or a psychiatric disorder. The two patients with absences as part of their idiopathic generalized epilepsies did not show retropulsive movements of the eyeballs or head. Although the eyelid movements in these absences were of a flickering kind and less rapid than in EMA, it can be difficult to distinguish these from eyelid myoclonus, and the diagnosis of EMA would be enhanced by stricter criteria as to what constitutes eyelid myoclonia, including electromyographic studies of the nature of the eyelid movements.

The ictal EEG changes in EMA generally showed faster spike or polyspike and wave than in typical or atypical absence seizures. Case 2 of the EMA group had a less characteristic ictal EEG with generalized slow activity rather than spike and wave. However, this patient was on sodium valporate and ethosuximide at the time of study, and the EEG may have been modified by this treatment. Photosensitivity was found in three of the five patients with EMA, but also occurred in the typical absence group. Spike-wave discharges and the occurrence of absences on slow eye closure is one of the characteristic features in EMA (Appleton *et al.* 1993). The effect of eye closure was not rigorously assessed in this series, as the cases were evaluated retrospectively. However, seizures may be precipitated by eye closure in other epilepsies with photosensitivity (Binnie *et al.* 1980).

The age of onset of seizures in the EMA group shows a wider range than in previous series, with onset apparently in mid teens in one case. However, this relatively late onset may reflect the difficulties of recognizing absences in young children, particularly when the seizures are closely related to environmental light stimulation and the children are erroneously considered to have mannerisms or other behavioural disorders. Diagnosis was delayed by a few years in most of the cases with EMA.

The majority of patients with EMA had generalized tonic-clonic seizures, although these were infrequent in all cases (Table 1). In contrast, only one patient had early morning myoclonic jerks, and this may be a useful discriminating feature between EMA and other types of idiopathic generalized epilepsy. The common occurrence of status in the EMA group is of interest, and has not been remarked upon in previous series. Three patients described frequent episodes of continuous absences and obtundation lasting for 24 or more hours, and in a fourth patient, very frequent seizures were considered to be contributing to poor performance on psychometric testing and low IQ. Absence status appears to be much less common in other types of idiopathic generalized epilepsy, with an incidence of 3 per cent in childhood absence epilepsy (Gibbs & Gibbs, 1952). The electrographic accompaniments of status in EMA·differ from those in other types of absence status, which is characterized by continuous spike and wave activity (Thomas *et al.* 1992). The episode of status documented on telemetry in case 4 showed discrete, albeit extremely frequent, bursts of spike-wave in association with brief absences.

Table 1. Clinical features in patients with EMA

Feature	Case 1	Case 2	Case 3	Case 4	Case 5
Onset * (yrs)	early childhood	9	8	15	3
GTCS	+	+	–	–	+
EM myoclonic jerks	–	+	–	–	–
Family history	+	–	+	–	+
Photosensitvity	+	+	+	–	NK
Status	–	?	+	+	+
Effective drugs	SVP+ESM	LTG+ESM	–	PHT+ESM	SVP

* = age at which absences first diagnosed; EM = early morning; + = present; – = absent, NK = not known (early EEGs unavailable), ? = no definite status (see text); SVP = sodium valproate; ESM = ethosuximide; LTG = lamotrigine; PHT = phenytoin

The most effective treatment for EMA has been suggested to be a combination of sodium valproate and ethosuximide (Appleton *et al.*, 1993). Effective regimens in this series were more varied, although in one case, seizures were virtually abolished when ethosuximide was added to sodium valporate. Sodium valporate alone produced a substantial reduction in seizures in one patient, who had not received this drug previously. The addition of lamotrigine to ethosuximide was highly effective in another case in whom sodium valproate had been associated with aggressive behaviour. Considerable improvement occurred in case 4 when ethosuximide was added to phenytoin. The fifth case had failed to respond to any treatment and was on no medication without apparent deterioration at the time of study.

Conclusion

Although none of the individual clinical features of the absence seizures of EMA is unique, the combination of brief absences, eyelid myoclonia and eyeball retropulsion with a normal neurological, intellectual and psychological state is sufficiently distinct to indicate that this is a discrete syndrome within the spectrum of idiopathic generalized epilepsies. Very few cases of this syndrome were identified amongst a large adult population of patients with epilepsy, suggesting that it is indeed rare. Absence seizures continue to occur with high frequency in adults with EMA, and status appears to be common, but considerable improvement in seizure control may be achieved using a combination of ethosuximide and other antiepileptic medications.

References

Appleton, R.E., Panayiotopoulos, C.P., Acomb B.A. & Beirne, M.(1993): Eyelid myoclonia with typical absences: an epilepsy syndrome. *J. Neurol. Neurosurg. Psychiatry* **56**, 1312–1316.

Binnie, C.D., Darby, C.E., de Korte, R.A. & Wilkins, A.J. (1980): Self-induction of epileptic seizures by eye-closure: incidence and recognition. *J. Neurol. Neurosurg. Psychiatry* **43**, 386–389.

Gibbs, F.A. & Gibbs, E.L. (1952): Petit mal. In: *Atlas of electroencephalography,* vol 2, eds F.A. Gibbs & E.L. Gibbs, pp. 55–65. Cambridge MA: Adison-Wesley Press Inc.

Thomas, P., Beaumonoir, A., Benton, P., Dolisi, C. & Chatel, M. (1992): "De novo" absence status of late onset: report of 11 cases. *Neurology* **42**, 104–110.

Eyelid Myoclonia with Absences, edited by J.S. Duncan and C.P. Panayiotopoulos
© 1996 John Libbey & Company Ltd, pp. 57–68.

Chapter 8

Eyelid myoclonia with absences in adults: clinical and EEG features

S. Giannakodimos and C.P. Panayiotopoulos

Department of Clinical Neurophysiology and Epilepsies, St. Thomas' Hospital, London, SE1 7EH UK

Eyelid myoclonia with absences (EMA) is a syndrome of idiopathic generalized epilepsy (IGE) not yet recognized by the International League Against Epilepsy although vividly described by Jeavons (1977; see chapter 2 this volume) and confirmed world-wide (Gobbi *et al.*, 1985; 1989; Dalla Bernardina *et al.*, 1989; Panayiotopoulos *et al.*, 1992; 1995; Appleton *et al.*, 1993; Covanis *et al.*, 1994; Panayiotopoulos, 1994a,b; 1995; 1996a,b,c; Appleton, 1995; Bianchi *et al.*, 1995; Isnard *et al.*, 1995; Giannakodimos & Panayiotopoulos, 1996).The patient reported by Radovici *et al.* in 1932 is probably the first documented case of EMA. EMA is a most distinct syndrome with a unique combination of characteristic clinico-EEG features which can be easily differentiated from other idiopathic generalized epilepsies syndromes (Panayiotopoulos, 1994a,b; 1995; 1996a,b,c). The key features are:

(a) Childhood onset of frequent, sometimes hundreds per day, brief seizures of eyelid myoclonia associated with absences. They are mainly induced by eye-closure, resist to treatment with sodium valproate alone, and persist in adult life where infrequent generalized tonic-clonic seizures are almost inevitable. Half of the patients also develop random myoclonic jerks of the limbs.

(b) Photosensitivity

(c) Characteristic, but not pathognomonic, ictal generalized discharges of mainly polyspikes and slow waves at 3-6 Hz which are brief (usually 3–4 s) and precipitated by eye-closure. They are eliminated in darkness (Panayiotopoulos, 1972; 1994b; 1996a,b).

We have studied the clinical and EEG features of EMA in 11 adult patients.

Methods and Patients

All patients with idiopathic generalized epilepsies and typical absences were classified according to strict clinical and video-EEG criteria (Panayiotopoulos *et al.*, 1995).Video-EEG after partial sleep deprivation followed by at least 30 minutes of video-EEG on awakening was often performed, especially if prolonged routine video-EEG had failed to record ictal phenomena.

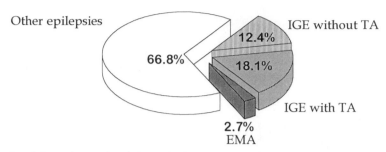

Prevalence of EMA amongst 410
patients older than 16 years of age

*Fig. 1. Prevalence of eyelid myoclonia (11 patients, 2.7 per cent) amongst 410
adult patients, older than 16 years of age; 136 (33.2 per cent) had idiopathic
generalized epilepsies and 85 (20.8 per cent) of them had absences.*

Our technique of intermittent photic stimulation, testing of fixation-off sensitivity and the effect of darkness on eye closure induced abnormalities have been detailed elsewhere (Panayiotopoulos, 1994a).

Strict selection criteria for EMA were applied. We have excluded photosensitive patients without eyelid myoclonia and patients with absences with eyelid fluttering (which is markedly different to the eyelid myoclonia of EMA) and who could be assigned to other syndromes of idiopathic generalized epilepsies. The mean follow-up period was 2 years (range: 1–5 years).

Results

Prevalence, sex, age, neurological state, and family history

Of 410 consecutive patients older than 16 years with epileptic seizures, 136 (33.2 per cent) had idiopathic generalized epilepsies. Of those with idiopathic generalized epilepsies, 85 (20.7 per cent of the total) had typical absences and 11 patients had EMA. Thus the prevalence of EMA was 2.7 per cent amongst all adult patients with epileptic disorders and 12.9 per cent amongst idiopathic generalized epilepsies and typical absences (Fig. 1).

All 11 patients were women of normal intelligence, and most were successful in their occupations. Their mean present age was 30.9 years (range: 16–45). Neurological examination and neuro-imaging with CT or MRI scan were normal in all patients. All but three patients had a family history of epileptic seizures. Two patients were sisters. Their only brother, who refused examination, was reported to have absences without apparent eyelid myoclonia, myoclonic jerks and generalized tonic-clonic seizures, while their mother had late onset, probably symptomatic, epileptic seizures (see also chapter 12). A brother of another patient was reported to have eyelid myoclonia-like movements without apparent epileptic seizures, and a first cousin was diagnosed as 'epileptic'.

Diagnosis and treatment on referral

Only one case was correctly diagnosed as EMA. Five patients were diagnosed as 'epilepsy', and five as 'absences', 'petit mal' or 'childhood absence epilepsy'. In seven patients, eyelid myoclonia was not appreciated as a seizure manifestation by the treating physicians.

Previous EEGs of all patients, recorded at various ages, demonstrated generalized spike/multiple

Age at Onset of Seizures

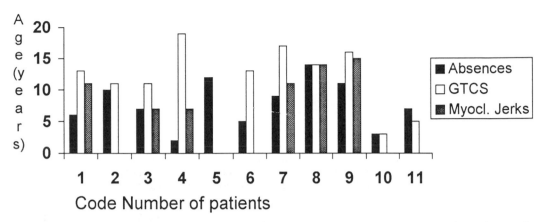

Fig. 2. Age at onset of eyelid myoclonia with absences, generalized tonic-clonic seizures and myoclonic jerks of the 11 patients with EMA.

spike and slow wave discharges and photosensitivity. Additional focal abnormalities occurred in four cases.

Two patients were not taking antiepileptic drugs. Four patients were on carbamazepine alone or in combination with ethosuximide or clonazepam; four were on sodium valproate in combination with either ethosuximide or phenobarbitone or primidone; and one was on ethosuximide, primidone and phenobarbitone.

Seizure types

Eyelid myoclonia with absence seizures

Eyelid myoclonia was the first symptom to attract attention, although it was often misinterpreted as a 'tic' or mannerism. It was described as rapid and brief eyelid flickering with upward jerking of the eyes and the head. Eyelid myoclonia occurred hundreds of times per day, often associated with moderate impairment of consciousness and was elicited by the sun or flickering lights. Onset was at a mean age of 7.8 ± 3.8 years (range 2–14 years, Fig. 2).

Absence status occurred in two patients, when ethosuximide was replaced by carbamazepine.

Generalized tonic-clonic seizures

Generalized tonic-clonic seizures occurred in all but the youngest patient. Onset was at 12.2 ± 5.0 years (range 3–19 years, Fig. 2). Generalized tonic-clonic seizures were usually infrequent, ranging from 1–12 per lifetime in all but two patients, in whom they were frequent generalized tonic-clonic seizures when they were not taking antiepileptic drugs or treated with inappropriate antiepileptic drugs. Generalized tonic-clonic seizures were mainly precipitated by sleep deprivation, fatigue, alcohol indulgence, inappropriate antiepileptic drugs, withdrawal of medication, flickering lights, or menstruation.

Myoclonic jerks

Eyelid myoclonia was often associated with retropulsive myoclonic jerking of the eyeballs and head. Infrequent myoclonic jerks of the upper limbs occurred in six patients either independently or together with the eyelid myoclonia.

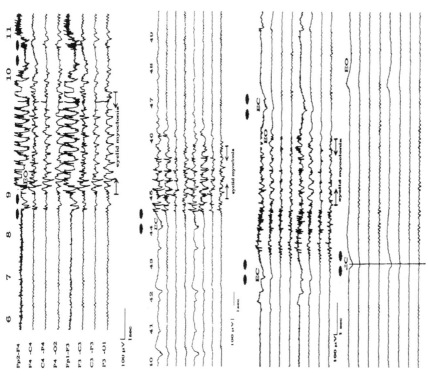

DARKNESS

Fig. 3. Video-EEG discharges associated with eyelid myoclonia with or without absences in three adult patients (three upper rows). Upper row: Immediately after closure on command indicated by two dark ovals on top of record, a brief generalized discharge occurred. After 1 s from onset eyelid myoclonia occurred. This was also associated with impairment of cognition as indicated by the delay in pronouncing the next number 10 on breath counting. Second row: Immediately after eye closure while the patient was counting, a brief absence occurred, clinically manifested with eyelid myoclonia and delay in counting (numbers annotated). Third row: Eyelid myoclonia on eye closure. Note the series of polyspikes during the first 2.5 seconds of the discharge. Eyelid myoclonia was seen only in the second part of the discharge; the latter shows polyspikes and slow waves at around 3 Hz. In all these three cases illustrated the seizures were induced by eye-closure. Darkness eliminated the discharges and seizures (lowest row).

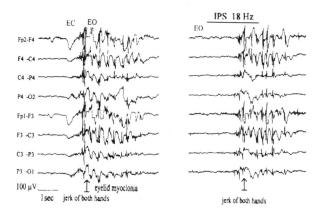

Fig. 4. Left: Eyelid myoclonia on eye closure, characterized by rhythmic jerks of the eyelids and the eyeballs with partial opening and upward deviation of the eyes starting 1 s after eye closure. A jerk of both hands occurred at the initial phase of the discharge, coinciding with a high amplitude polyspike and slow wave complex. Right: photoparoxysmal response during intermittent photic stimulation, on eye opening. Clinically, only a single jerk of both hands was recorded.

Partial seizures

Partial seizures did not occur. However, one of the patients had a history of benign childhood epilepsy with centrotemporal spikes before developing EMA. Her case was the subject of an earlier report because of the catamenial variation of her absences and the aggravating effect of progesterone (Grunewald *et al.*, 1992).

Photosensitivity

All patients were photosensitive. In eight of them photosensitivity started in childhood, as early as 3 years of age. However, clinical and EEG photosensitivity declined with age. At present, three out of the 11 patients have only minor posterior abnormalities induced by the intermittent photic stimulation and one has a normal EEG.

Self-induction

None of our patients was known or suspected by relatives or friends to have self-induced seizures (see chapter 11).

Video-EEG: ictal clinical and EEG manifestations

All 11 patients had at least one video-EEG, and seven had one to four additional video-EEGs during sleep and on awakening. Ictal phenomena were recorded in all but one patient who had a normal EEG. The ictal clinical and EEG manifestations were as follows:

Eyelid myoclonia with absences

This is the most typical seizure type in EMA and was recorded in five patients (Fig. 3). The seizure started with eyelid myoclonia consisting of fast (4–6 Hz), small range myoclonic jerks of the eyelids with simultaneous vertical jerking and upward deviation of the eyes. The eyes remained in a

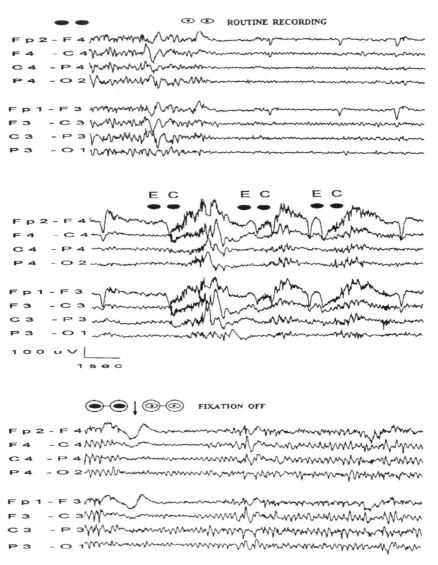

Fig. 5. Video-EEG recording of a female patient with EMA. She had onset of eyelid myoclonia in late childhood. Onset of generalized tonic-clonic seizures was at age of 11 years. She had only three generalized tonic-clonic seizures in her life which were precipitated by TV viewing (more details and her family history in chapter 12). She was clinically and EEG photosensitive. In addition, her EEGs in an illuminated room showed continuous generalized theta activity intermixed with sharp waves and spikes as long as the eyes remained closed. Total darkness and elimination of fixation inhibited eye closure discharges but facilitated 'eyes closed' abnormalities. Thus this patient had both photosensitive and fixation-off characteristics.

Upper: Recording with light-on. The 'eye-closed' abnormalities are eliminated when she opens her eyes.
Middle: Eye-closure induced abnormalities associated with brief eyelid myoclonia.
Lower: Recording in darkness. There is only a brief attenuation of the abnormalities on eyes closed but soon after the EEG is dominated by generalized theta activity intermixed with sharp waves and spikes as seen in eyes-closed conditions.

semi-open position during the ictus irrespective of whether the seizure started on eyes closed, opened or on eye closure. This is probably due to a tonic contraction of the eyelid elevators during the seizure. Occasionally, there were simultaneous myoclonic jerks of the eyebrows or the head. In addition, in one patient, eyelid myoclonia was associated with deviation of the eyes and the head to the right, and in another patient with jerks of both hands (Figure 4). Absences occurred only as part of this type of seizure, while eyelid myoclonia continued. Absences were usually mild, manifested with abnormalities of breath counting. Automatisms were never observed.

The ictal EEG showed generalized discharges of mainly polyspikes and polyspike/slow waves at 3-6 Hz with a mean duration of 3.2 ± 1.2 s (range 1.5–9.0 s) (Fig. 3). Only one seizure lasted more than 6 s. The onset of the discharges was simultaneous or preceding, never occurring after, the onset of the eyelid phenomena.

Eyelid myoclonia without absences

Eyelid myoclonia, often associated with myoclonic jerks of the eyes, head or other muscles but without discernible absences, occurred in all five patients described above and in an additional three patients. The ictal EEG mainly showed generalized polyspike discharges of brief (1–2 s) duration (Figs. 3 and 4).

Milder manifestations consisting of brief ($1 \leq$ s), abortive eyelid myoclonia with eyelid tremor-like jerks or eyelid fluttering also occurred either with EEG accompaniments (all but one patient) or without apparent EEG changes (all but two patients). When EEG changes were absent, eyelid manifestations were usually extremely mild. However, three patients also had infrequent eyelid myoclonia-like movements without EEG changes. Additionally, two patients also had rare and mild jerks of the head or hands during intermittent photic stimulation without EEG accompaniments.

None of our patients showed repetitive full-scale eye-blinking without EEG discharges, as described in patients attempting seizure self-induction (see chapter 10).

Video-EEG: precipitating factors

Eye closure

Eye closure was the most potent precipitating factor in the 10 patients with abnormal EEGs. Brief ($6 \leq$ s), high voltage generalized multiple spike and slow wave discharges appeared within 0.5–2 s after closing the eyes in an illuminated recording room. The eye closure-related discharges were associated with all the various clinical manifestations already detailed but could also occur without discernible clinical symptoms. Total darkness eliminated the eye closure-induced EEG discharges in all 10 patients (Fig. 3).

Fixation-off sensitivity

One patient (case 2 in Giannakodimos & Panayiotopoulos, 1996) was of particular interest in that, in addition to eye closure related EEG abnormalities she showed continuous generalized theta activity intermixed with sharp waves and spikes as long as the eyes remained closed (Fig. 5). Total darkness and elimination of fixation inhibited eye closure discharges but facilitated 'eyes closed' abnormalities. Thus, this patient had both photosensitive and fixation-off characteristics (Panayiotopoulos, 1994a; 1996a,b).

Intermittent photic stimulation

Six patients had photoconvulsive responses (Fig. 4); one refused testing because of a high degree of photosensitivity, three showed mild posterior abnormalities, and one had a normal EEG.

Overbreathing, sleep and awakening

Overbreathing increased the epileptiform discharges in all patients with abnormal EEGs. Sleep increased the polyspike and slow wave discharges in four patients, reduced them in two and had no effect in one. The discharges during sleep were shorter (1–2 s) and unaccompanied by discernible clinical manifestations of any type, even in those patients with numerous seizures during alertness. EEG and clinical manifestations were consistently deteriorated after awakening.

Treatment

The recognition of EMA resulted in appropriate modification of treatment in nearly all patients. Presently, eight patients are treated with sodium valproate, either alone or in combination with ethosuximide, clonazepam or primidone. One patient is only on clobazam and two others are not taking antiepileptic drugs. Eyelid myoclonia persists in nine patients, although absences have improved in all patients taking antiepileptic drugs and none have had generalized tonic-clonic seizures.

Discussion

EMA is a predominantly myoclonic syndrome, mainly characterized by localized eyelid myoclonus. Typical absences are part of this type of seizure, they do not occur without eyelid myoclonia, and they have no similarities to the absences occurring in other idiopathic generalized epilepsies syndromes (see chapter 6).

This study in adult patients showed that eyelid myoclonia is not only the characteristic symptom of EMA but also the most resistant to treatment, occurring many times per day, often without apparent absences and even without demonstrable photosensitivity. Eyelid myoclonia is mainly induced by eye-closure, is enhanced by the presence of flashing or stable light and is eliminated by darkness (Panayiotopoulos, 1994a; 1996a,b). The combination of photosensitive epilepsy and fixation-off sensitivity, which are two apparently antagonistic conditions, in the same patient is an extremely interesting situation which is difficult to explain, and should be attributed to the functional properties of the occipital lobes (Wilkins, 1995). Conversion of photosensitive to fixation-off sensitive epilepsy has been previously reported (Panayiotopoulos, 1989; 1996b).

It was exceptional for any of our patients not to demonstrate eyelid myoclonia on follow-up, even long after other seizure types had been completely controlled. This may imply considerable problems for situations, such as driving, in which legal requirements specify a seizure-free state.

Eyelid myoclonia alone is not sufficient to characterize the syndrome of EMA as it may also be seen in other epileptic conditions, mainly cryptogenic and symptomatic (see also chapter 6). Generalized tonic-clonic seizures, although usually infrequent, are probably inevitable in adult life, and myoclonic jerks of the limbs may occur in half of the patients. A family history of epilepsies is common (see chapter 13).

The following definition for the syndrome of EMA is proposed (Giannakodimos & Panayiotopoulos, 1996):

EMA is an idiopathic myoclonic epileptic syndrome which is genetically determined. It is mainly manifested by eyelid myoclonia which in the same patient may occur alone or proceed to an absence. Eyelid myoclonia consists of marked, rhythmic and fast jerks of the eyelids, often with upward jerking of the eyes and the head. There is probably an associated tonic component of the involved muscles. Impairment of consciousness occurs when seizures are longer, but it is of mild or moderate severity and is not associated with automatisms. Absence seizures do not occur without eyelid myoclonia. Mild eyelid myoclonia can occur without absences, especially in adult and treated patients, and may also occur without EEG discharges. Seizures are brief (3–6 s) and occur mainly after eye closure. All patients are photosensitive, but photosensitivity decreases with age. Onset is usually in early childhood. Generalized tonic-clonic seizures are probably inevitable but tend to be infrequent, often precipitated by flickering lights, sleep deprivation, fatigue and alcohol indulgence. Myoclonic jerks of the limbs occur in 50 per cent of the patients, but are infrequent and random.. Eyelid myoclonia is resistant to treatment and may be lifelong, but the associated impairment of consciousness may become less frequent and less severe with age.

The ictal EEG manifestations consist of brief (1–6 s) generalized polyspikes/slow waves at 3–6 Hz, which are more likely to occur after eye closure in an illuminated room. Total darkness abolishes the eye closure related EEG abnormalities. Eye-closure manifestations may persist without photosensitivity. Photoconvulsive responses are recorded from all untreated young patients.

Differential diagnosis of typical absences and syndromes of idiopathic generalized epilepsies (Panayiotopoulos, 1996c)

The differential diagnosis of typical absences with severe impairment of consciousness in children from other type of seizures is relatively easy and confirmed with EEG with 3–4 Hz generalized spike/polyspike and slow wave. Typical absences may be missed in babies if they are not associated with myoclonic components (Aicardi, 1995). In EMA, the eyelid myoclonia predominates and absences may be missed; they are often misdiagnosed as tic or mannerism. The diagnosis of typical absences in adults is even more difficult. In our studies, typical absences had frequently been unrecognized for years or misdiagnosed as complex partial seizures (Panayiotopoulos *et al.*, 1992; 1995) because they are usually mild and may even, although exceptionally, be associated with derealization and fear.

Most physicians are unfamiliar with the syndromic classification of absence epilepsies and great diversity of opinion exists amongst experts about their definitive criteria (Panayiotopoulos, 1994b; 1996c). For teaching purposes we found it useful to start the differential diagnosis of these syndromes (Duncan & Panayiotopoulos, 1995) from the most easy to diagnose.

The diagnosis of EMA is the easiest of all as it is betrayed by the characteristic eyelid myoclonia. However, eyelid myoclonia should not be confused with the rhythmic or random closing of the eyes which is often seen in other forms of absence syndromes (chapter 6). Furthermore, their very short duration, the photosensitivity and the precipitation of eyelid myoclonia absences by eye-closure as well as the predominantly polyspike-wave EEG discharges make EMA a syndrome which should not be misdiagnosed. The problem is with eyelid myoclonia and photosensitivity in cryptogenic or symptomatic epilepsies which are associated with learning difficulties and often behavioural problems. The latter are incompatible with EMA which is a form of idiopathic generalized epilepsies.

Equally easy to diagnose is the syndrome of myoclonic absence epilepsy with the characteristically rhythmic myoclonic jerks mainly of the upper extremities. Again, it is divided into idiopathic and cryptogenic/symptomatic.

Perioral myoclonia with absences, in our experience, is often erroneously diagnosed as motor partial epilepsy in adults and childhood absence epilepsy in children. A clear history of marked perioral jerking is often obtained if a detailed history is taken. However, in most cases video-EEG is essential to confirm the diagnosis; this investigation is a requirement for full evaluation of both children and adults with typical absences. Video-EEG recordings demonstrate the rhythmic jerks of the perioral and/or jaw muscles coinciding with the polyspikes of the spike-wave complexes. Onset of generalized tonic-clonic seizures before or at the same age as typical absences, the brief duration of absences, the EEG irregularities and the occurrence of absence status are useful clinical indicators in favour of perioral myoclonia with absences and against childhood or juvenile absence epilepsy.

Juvenile myoclonic epilepsy should not be difficult to diagnose if fully developed at late adolescence and adulthood (Panayiotopoulos *et al.*, 1989). Myoclonic jerks on awakening, obtained through a skilful interview with the patient, are the hallmark of the disease. However, one third of the patients also have absences at the onset of the disease. We have extensively studied the clinico-video-EEG characteristics of typical absences in juvenile myoclonic epilepsy (Panayiotopoulos *et al.*, 1989a,b). When typical absences of juvenile myoclonic epilepsy start in childhood or early adolescence their differentiation from childhood absence epilepsy and juvenile absene epilepsy is difficult, but essential for prognostic reasons. The absences of juvenile myoclonic epilepsy are usually simple (with no automatisms, localised or limb jerks), the impairment of consciousness only occasionally may be severe (but not as much as in childhood absence epilepsy or juvenile absence epilepsy) and the EEG discharges are often fragmented with Ws (multiple spikes having the appearance of compressed Ws).

In adolescents, the differential diagnosis may be difficult between juvenile absence epilepsy and juvenile myoclonic epilepsy. However, absences are the major problem in the former (more frequent and with severe impairment of consciousness) but not in the latter, (in which typical absences are often so mild as to be not easily discernible). However, it should be emphasized that video-EEG studies, of patients with juvenile myoclonic epilepsy having typical absences in childhood or early adolescence are needed for the validation of these statements. Irrespective of the results of these studies which are awaited, it is not justifiable to speak about patients with childhood or juvenile absence epilepsy developing juvenile myoclonic epilepsy. It is juvenile myoclonic epilepsy which starts with typical absences in childhood or early adolescence. A child with frequent typical absences, later developing and generalized tonic-clonic seizures, does not have childhood absence epilepsy evolving to juvenile myoclonic epilepsy: he has absences as the first manifestation of juvenile myoclonic epilepsy with onset in childhood. In the majority of these patients with juvenile myoclonic epilepsy starting with typical absences in childhood, video-EEG studies will clearly differentiate them form the typical absences of childhood absence epilepsy. However, there may be cases in which their differentiation is difficult and juvenile myoclonic epilepsy will not be diagnosed until many years after with the appearance of myoclonic jerks and generalized tonic-clonic seizures.

In childhood absence epilepsy and juvenile absence epilepsy, typical absences are the main, the most disturbing and the most characteristic type of seizures. Childhood absence epilepsy is manifested with typical absences only, which are age related. There are no myoclonic jerks, no generalized tonic-clonic seizures and no photosensitivity. The impairment of consciousness is more severe than in any other syndrome and the EEG discharge is harmonious, with no polyspikes or fragmentation. Further studies are needed for the precise identification of the ictal clinical manifestations but consistent myoclonic jerks, localized or generalized, should raise suspicion against such a diagnosis which, by definition should define a self-limited disease in childhood.

Juvenile absence epilepsy is the only syndrome in which the ictal manifestations of typical absences many clinical and EEG similarities to those of childhood absence epilepsy (Panayiotopoulos *et al.*, 1989a). However, they are milder, less frequent and longer than those of childhood absence epilepsy, although these differences are often subtle and not sufficient for a confident diagnosis. Juvenile absence epilepsy is also characterised by typical absences which are severe and persist in adult life, they start towards late childhood to adolescence and are often associated with infrequent generalized tonic-clonic seizures and sporadic, infrequent myoclonic jerks. There is no suggestion of eyelid, perioral or limb myoclonia.

Acknowledgements

We thank the British Telecom Charitable Organisation and Special Trustees of St. Thomas' Hospital for financial support of our studies on the classification of epilepsies.

References

Aicardi, J. (1995): Typical absences in the first two years of life. In: *Typical absences and related epileptic syndromes,* edited by J.S. Duncan and C.P. Panayiotopoulos. pp. 284-288. London: Churchill Livingstone.

Appleton, R.E. (1995): Eyelid myoclonia with absences. In: Typical absences and related epileptic syndrome, ed. J.S. Duncan & C.P. Panyiotopoulis. pp. 213–20. London: Churchill Livingstone.

Appleton, R.E., Panayiotopoulos, C.P., Acomb, B.A. & Beirne, M. (1993): Eyelid myoclonia with typical absences: an epilepsy syndrome. *J. Neurol. Neurosurg. Psychiatry* **56**, 1312–1316

Bianchi, A. and the Italian League Against Epilepsy (1995): Studies of concordance of syndromes in families with absence epilepsies. In: *Typical absences and related epileptic syndromes,* edited by J.S. Duncan and C.P. Panayiotopoulos. pp. 328–337. London: Churchill Livingstone.

Covanis, A., Skiadas, C., Loli, N., Ioannidou, A., Lada, C. & Theodorou, V. (1994): Eyelid myoclonia with absences. *Epilepsia* **35**, (suppl. 7): 13.

Dalla Bernardina, B., Sgro, V., Fontana., E. *et al.* (1989): Eyelid myoclonia with absences. In: *Reflex seizures and reflex epilepsies,* eds. A. Beaumanoir, H. Gastaut, and R. Naquet, pp. 193-200. Geneva: Medecine et Hygiene.

Duncan, J.S. & Panayiotopoulos, C.P. (1995): *Typical absences and related epileptic syndromes.* London: Churchill Livingstone.

Giannakodimos, S. & Panayiotopolous, C.P. (1996): Eyelid myoclonia with absences in adults: a clinical and video-EEG study. *Epilepsia* **37**, 36–44.

Gobbi, G., Tinuper, P., Tassinari, C.A. *et al.* (1985): Le mioclonie palpebrali con assenza alla chiusura degli occhi. *Boll. Lega. It. Epil.* **51/52**, 225–226.

Gobbi, G., Bruno, L., Mainetti, A., Parmegianni, A., Tullini, A., Salvi, F., Tassinari, C.A., Santanelli, P., Bureau, M., Dravet, C.H. & Roger, J. (1989): Eye-closure seizures. In: *Reflex seizures and reflex epilepsies,* eds. A. Beaumanoir, H. Gastaut, and R. Naquet, pp. 181–191. Geneva: Medecine et Hygiene.

Grünewald, R.A., Aliberti, V. & Panayiotopoulos, C.P. (1992): Exacerbation of typical absence seizures by progesterone. *Seizure* **1**, 137–138.

Isnard, H., Badinand-Hubert, N., Keo-Kosal, P., Revol, M. (1995): Twenty-one cases of eyelid myoclonia with absences. *Epilepsia* **36**, (suppl. 3) S200.

Jeavons, P.M. (1977): Nosological problems of myoclonic epilepsies in childhood and adolescence. *Dev. Med. Child. Neurol.* **19**, 3–8.

Panayiotopoulos, C.P. (1972): A study of photosensitive epilepsy with particular reference to occipital spikes induced by intermittent photic stimulation. Ph.D. Thesis. Univeristy of Aston Birmingham.

Panayiotopoulos, C.P. (1979): Conversion of photosensitive to scotosensitive epilepsy. *Neurology* **30**, 1550–1555.

Panayiotopoulos, C.P. (1994a): Fixation-off-sensitive epilepsies: clinical and EEG characteristics. In: *Epileptic seizures and syndromes,* ed., P. Wolf, pp. 55–65. London: John Libbey.

Panayiotopoulos, C.P. (1994b): The clinical spectrum of typical absence seizures and absence epilepsies. In: *Idiopathic generalized epilepsies: clinical, experimental and genetic aspects,* eds. A. Malafosse, P. Genton, E. Hirsch, C. Marescaux, D. Broglin, R. & Bernasconi R., pp. 75–85. London: John Libbey.

Panayiotopoulos C.P. (1995): Typical absences are syndrome-related. In: *Typical absences and related epileptic syndromes,* edited by J.S. Duncan and C.P. Panayiotopoulos., pp. 304–314. London: Churchill Livingstone.

Panayiotopoulos, C.P. (1996a): Epilepsies characterised by seizures with specific modes of precipitation (Reflex epilepsies). In: *Childhood epilepsy,* ed. S. Wallace, pp. 355–375. London: Chapman & Hall.

Panayiotopoulos, C.P. (1996b): Fixation-off sensitive, scotosensitive and other visual-related sensitive epilepsies. In: *Reflex epilepsies,* eds. S. Zifkin *et al.* New York: Raven Press (in press).

Panayiotopoulos, C.P. (1996c): Absence epilepsies: childhood, juvenile and myoclonic absence epilepsy, eyelid myoclonia with absences and other related epileptic syndromes with typical absence seizures. In: *Epilepsy: a comprehensive textbook,* eds, J.E. Engel & T.A. Pedley. (Volume 3, in press). New York: Raven Press.

Panayiotopoulos, C.P., Obeid, T. & Waheed, G. (1989a): Differentiation of typical absences in epileptic syndromes. A video EEG study of 224 seizures in 20 patients. *Brain* **112**, 1039–1056.

Panayiotopoulos, C.P., Obeid, T. & Waheed, G. (1989b): Absences in JME: a clinical and video-electroencephalographic study. *Ann. Neurol.* **25**, 391–397.

Panayiotopoulos, C.P., Chroni, E., Daskalopoulos, C., Baker, A., Rowlinson, S., Walsh, P. (1992): Typical absence seizures in adults: clinical, EEG, video-EEG findings and diagnostic/syndromic considerations. *J. Neurology, Neurosurgery and Psychiatry* **55**, 1002–1008.

Panayiotopoulos, C.P., Giannakodimos, S. & Chroni, E. (1995): Typical absences in adults. In: *Typical absences and related epileptic syndromes,* eds. J.S.Duncan and C.P.Panayiotopoulos. pp. 289–299. London: Churchill Livingstone.

Radovici, A., Misirliou, V. & Gluckman, M.L. (1932): Epilepsie reflexe provoque par excitations optiques des rayons solaires. *Revue Neurologique.* **1,** 1305–1307.

Wilkins, A.J. (1995): Towards an understanding of reflex epilepsy and the absence. In: *Typical absences and related epileptic syndromes*, eds. J.S. Duncan and C.P. Panayiotopoulos. pp. 195–205. Churchill Livingstone: London.

Eyelid Myoclonia with Absences, edited by J.S. Duncan and C.P. Panayiotopoulos
© 1996 John Libbey & Company Ltd, pp. 69–76.

Chapter 9

Eye closure and EEG abnormalities, darkness, fixation-off and photosensitivity

G.F.A. Harding

Department of Vision Sciences, Clinical Neurophysiology Unit, Aston University, Aston Triangle, Birmingham, B4 7ET, UK

In 1964 Pantelakis *et al.* (1962) reported that abnormalities evoked by intermittent photic stimulation were more likely when the patients' eyes were closed than when they were open. Many previous studies (Bickford *et al.*, 1953), Melsen, 1959, Pallis & Lewis, 1961 had produced similar findings and later authors such as Brausch & Ferguson (1965), Troupin (1966), Bickford & Klass (1969) and Kooi (1971) confirmed these earlier results and suggested a variety of explanations. Some suggested that the eylids acted as a red filter or that they diffused light, increasing the area of the retina illuminated, and Bickford & Klass (1969) suggested that the reduction in visual pattern input may play a part in these increased abnormalites. A similar loss of visual attention was suggested by Pantelakis *et al.* (1962).

Contrary to the above reports, Jeavons *et al.* (1966) found that patients were much more sensitive in the eyes-open than in the eyes-closed state and recognized that many previous investigators had made no distinction between the act of eye closure and the state of eyes-closed. It is well known that many patients show spontaneous spike and wave discharges immediately following eye closure (Bickford & Klass, 1969; Atzev 1962; Green, 1966 and 1968; Jeavons *et al.* 1966; Kooi, 1971). Atzev (1962) had reported that 7 per cent of 402 patients who had EEG abnormalites evoked by intermittent photic stimulation showed this spontaneous abnormality in their resting EEG.

Our study of 454 patients with photosensitive epilepsy showed that of 253 patients with abnormalities in their EEG, 90 (36 per cent) had shown spike and wave discharges on eye closure (Jeavons & Harding, 1975); because of this high association with photosensitive epilepsy such a discharge in the resting EEG indicates a high probability that abnormality will be evoked by IPS (Harding & Jeavons, 1994).

In defining these spike-wave discharges which occur following eye closure it is important to realize that the discharges usually involve all regions (Fig. 1) and must be distinguished from the physiological resonse to eye closure consisting of high amplitude slow waves confined to the

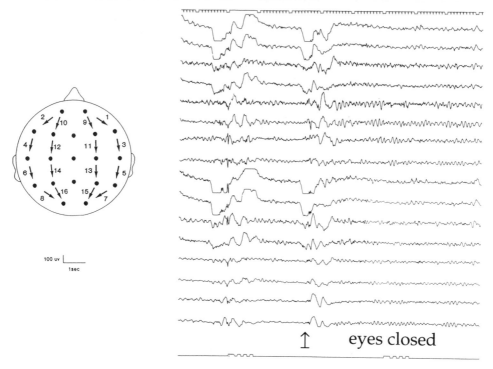

100 uv

1sec

↑   eyes closed

Fig. 1. Shows a paroxysmal discharge consisting of spikes and waves occurring at the time of an eye blink and then when the eyes are closed. It can be seen that both anterior and posterior regions of the brain are involved the spikes appearing both occipitally and frontally. The discharges occur immediately after a blink or immediately after eye closure. These discharges occurred in the resting record without stimulation.

posterior regions, often seen in children. Other physiological phenomena such as the 'squeak' activity seen on eye closure in which faster frequencies of alpha activity are present must be carefully differentiated (Storm Van Leeuwen & Bekkering, 1958).

Our initial studies therefore separated the eyes-closed state from the act of eye closure. In addition, we had standardized the technique whereby intermittent photic stimulation was performed using Grass PS22 photic stimulator at intensity 2 set at a distance of 30 cm from the eyes under conditions of normal room illumination but with all external light excluded. The abnormal response was defined as a photoparoxysmal response which was bilateral and recorded simultaneously in all areas of the scalp and consisted of a spike and wave discharge with a slow wave component often at 3.5 Hz (Fig. 2.) The results of our original study are contained in Table 1. When the state of eyes-closed was separated from the act of eye closure it was clearly apparent that responses were more prevalent to intermittent photic stimulation with the eyes open than with the eyes closed. The nine patients who showed sensitivity to eye-closure alone were of course the only ones who were tested under that condition since it was our practice at that time not to use eye closure during intermittent photic stimulation unless we had previously shown that there was no abnormality elicited in both the eyes-open or the eyes-closed state. There is therefore no doubt that eye closure during intermittent photic stimulation is the most provocative condition and this would explain the findings by other investigators.

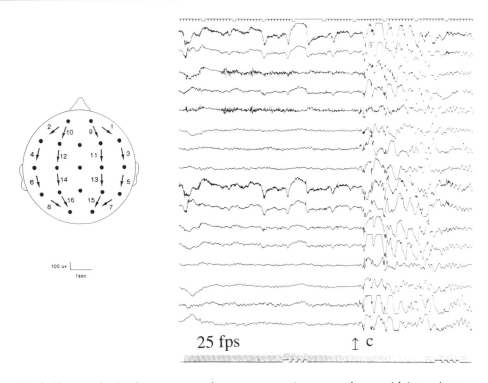

25 fps   ↑ C

Fig. 2. Shows a classic photoparoxysmal response occurring on eye closure with intermittent photic stimulation at 25 f.p.s. The discharge consists of irregular 3 Hz spike and wave activity and it should be noted that discharge terminates whilst stimulation continues, indicating that the act of eye closure is more provocative than the eyes-closed condition in which only the normal background activity is seen.

Table 1. Prevalence of photoparoxysmal discharges under various eye conditions in photosensitive epilepsy

Eye state	All cases (n = 292)	
	n	**%**
Eyes open only	176	60
Eyes open > closed	82	28
Eyes closed only	5	2
Eyes closed > eyes open	14	5
Eyes open = eyes closed	6	2
Eye closure only	9	3

As was pointed out earlier, 90 of our 454 patients showed spike and wave discharges in the resting record following eye closure. This known association with photosensitivuty has been studied in detail by Panayiotopoulous (1974, 1981 and 1989) using some of our original patients as well as some others, and he carried out detailed studies on eye closure abnormalities. In a study of six patients with abnormalities in their basic EEG elicted by eye closure he showed that no abnormal responses could be produced by eye closure in darkness, although transient passive eye closure in illumination would produce abnormality. More recently he also reported fixation-off sensitivity in which patients produce paroxysmal EEG features in the eyes closed condition which may progress to epileptic seizures (Panayiotopoulous, 1989). The paroxysmal activity usually consists of bilateral

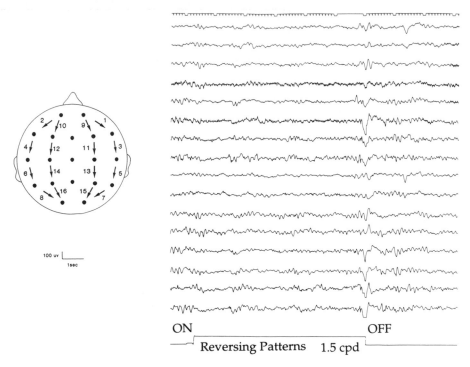

100 uv

1sec

ON _____ OFF

Reversing Patterns   1.5 cpd

Fig. 3. Shows a fixation-off response occurring during pattern stimulation without any intermittent photic stimulation. The subject was seated 1 metre from the stimulus which consisted of a video monitor on which which contrasting black and white bars at 1.5 c.p.d. were presented. The pattern was oscillating and appeared out of a neutral equal luminance background and disappeared into the same background at the termination of the stimulus. It should be noted that the discharge occured only at the moment the stimulus was turned off.

spike and wave complexes confined to the occipital regions, only seen in the eyes-closed condition, and blocks or attenuates when the eyes are opened. Such discharges may occur in eyes-open condition when there is absence of central vision and fixation. Patients with these abnormalities may be separated from those with photosensitivity by the fact that eye-closed EEG abnormalities continue in total darkness and remain if the eyes are open in total darkness. Occassionaly a variety of fixation-off responses is seen in patients who are undergoing pattern sensitivity testing (Fig. 3). Under these circumstances when a pattern which is either reversing or stationary appears out of a neutral equiluminant backround and then disappears into the neutral backround again the only abnormal discharges are elicited by the change from the pattern to the diffused background.

Scotosensitive or scotogenic seizures may be part of this fixation-off syndrome (Panayiotopoulos, 1989). Scotogenic seizures were first described by Gumnit *et al.* (1965), who pointed out that these seizures were uniquely inhibited by the establishment of pattern vision, though Beaumanoir *et al.* (1989) and Gastaut (1982, 1985) and others have reported the existence of these seizures in children and adolescence and have pointed out that these patients frequently show occipital foci which can be triggered by the passage from dark to light or light to dark (Gastaut, 1985). Panayiotopoulos (1979) reported the case of a patient who changed from phtosensitivity to scotosensitivity. Beaumanoir *et al.* (1989) indicated that in these patients the discharge may be precipitated by terminating periods of intermittent photic stimulation. From this point of view, therefore, they appear to be part of the fixation-off syndrome and represent a different form of visual sensitivity. Certainly any such

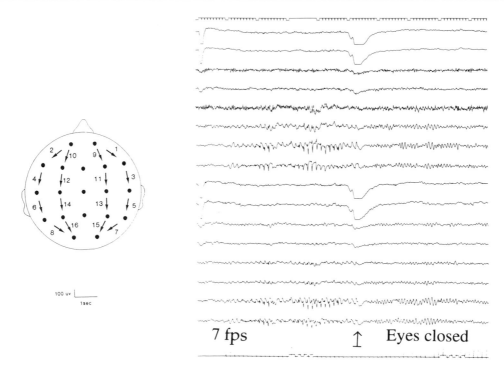

Fig. 4. Shows occipital spikes in response to intermittent photic stimulation stimulation at 7 f.p.s. The spikes occur at the same rate as the flash and are electronegative at the occiput. They are entirely confined to posterior regions and cease when the eyes are closed.

sensitivity that is demonstrated by these patients should be in the form of abnormal responses seen either in posterior regions or as a photoparoxysmal response produced by stopping the train of intermittent photic stimuli.

Although there is evidence that many patients are both photo- and pattern-sensitive there is also evidence that pattern sensitivity my occur in patients in the absence of photosensitivity (Harding *et al.*, 1994). Indeed in many previous studies (Harding & Jeavons, 1994) we have also demonstrated that the superimposition of a pattern on the diffused illuminated screen of the photic stimulator increases the probability of producing abnormal discharges. In addition, we have also demonstrated that such a pattern markedly increases the probability of inducing occipital spikes (Harding & Dimitrakoudi, 1977).

Occipital spikes are defined as abnormalities evoked in the occipital regions by intermittent photic stimulation. At low flash rates, they occur at the same rate as the flash and are always electronegative to the occipital electrode (Fig. 4). When they occur in isolation from photoparoxysmal responses they do not necessarily indicate epilepsy (Maheshwari & Jeavons, 1975). Of a total of 280 cases investigated in our original series, 179 (64 per cent) showed occipital spikes. They do not represent an exaggerated visual evoked potential since the negative occipital spike occurs on the descending wave of the second positive component of the visual evoked potential (Harding & Dimitrakoudi, 1977). Occipital spikes are always clearly enhanced if a pattern is superimposed over the diffused photo-stimulator (Harding & Jeavons, 1994). Occipital spikes represent evidence of hyperexcitability of the visual cortex (Harding & Jeavons, 1994). Spikes confined to the occipital regions, when they are present and of high amplitude, may be associated with a subjective sensation (Fig. 5). Further, the occipital spike may frequently act as a precursor to a photoparoxysmal

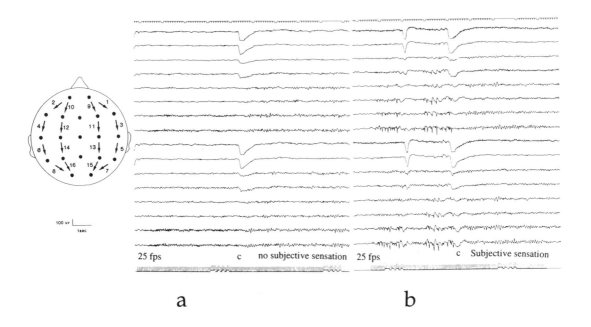

Fig. 5. Shows occipital spikes only produced during intermittent photic stimulation (IPS) using a photo stimulator which has a superimposed grid (Harding & Jeavons, 1994), trace (b). In traces at the same IPS but without grid and with only a diffuser there are no occipital spikes, trace (a). In this patient the occipital spikes were accompanied by a subjective sensation.

response. This is often seen as the flash rate of the photic stimulus is increased so that occipital spikes occur in isolation at low flash rates, and then as a precursor to the photoparoxysmal discharge at higher flash rates.

Photosensitive epilepsy requires the presence of a hyperexcitable visual cortex as well as a low convulsive threshold. Sodium valproate is highly effective in patients with photosensitive epilepsy and abolishes the photoparoxysmal response but never affects the presence of occipital spikes (Herrick & Harding 1980). Under these circumstances patients continue to show occipital spikes but no longer have convultions when viewing television with either broadcast material or video material.

Using our provocative techniques of intermittent photic stimulation with a superimposed pattern a large perenctage of patients show occipital spikes – 86 per cent of 38 patients in one study – and none of these patients showed eye closure abnormalities. Of 39 of our current patients who did show eye closure abnormalities in the resting EEG only five showed occipital spikes (Table 2).

Table 2. Association of occipital spikes with normal presponses to eye clsure in the basic EEG

Basic EEG	Occipital spikes present	No occipital spikes
Eye closure abnormal	5	34
Eye closure normal	49	25

Significance = $P < 0.001$ (X^2 tail test).

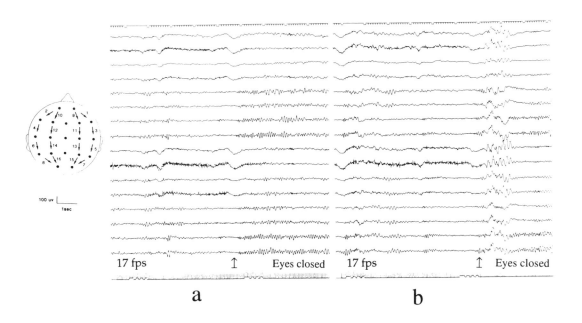

Fig. 6. Effect of eye closure during intermittent photic stimulation either with a grid superimposed (a) or with a simple diffuser (b). It can be seen that no clear abnormalities are evoked during (a), and when the eyes are closed during the intermittent photic stimulation only alpha activity is seen. In trace (b) eye closure during diffused intermittent photic stimulation produces a clear photoparoxysmal response which terminates within 1.5 s of eye closure even though the intermittent photic stimulation continued.

Taken as a whole these findings suggest that patients with eye closure abnormalities either on intermittent photic stimulation or in the resting record may represent a separate subgroup of patients and that the reduction in visual pattern input first suggested by Bickford & Klass (1969) may be true for these patients. Indeed when such patients do show eye closure abnormalities it is quite often the case that diffused intermittent photic stimulation may be more provocative than patterned stimulation (Fig. 6). This would therefore suggest that the hyperexcitable visual cortex, – as represented by occipital spikes, – giving rise to secondary generaliztion in photosensitive epilepsy could be different subgroup of photosensitive from patients who show either fixation-off, eye closure or so called scotosensitive epilepsy. Indeed this latter group of patients, like the EMA group, may well not have visual cortex which responds with hyperexcitability to supranormal stimulation, such as flashed-on patterns.

References

Atzev, E. (1962): The effect of closing the eyes upon epileptic activity. *J. Electroencephalogr. Clin. Neurophysiol.* **14,** 561.

Beaumanoir, A., Capizzi, G., Nahory, A. & Yousfi, Y. (1989): Fixation-off sensitive epilepsies. In: Beaumanoir, A. Gastaut, H., Naquet, R., eds *Reflex seizures and reflex epilepsies.* International Symposium on Reflex Seizures and Reflex Epilepsies, Genève, June 1988. Geneva: Médecine & Hygiène pp. 219–227.

Bickford, R.G., Daly, D. & Keith, H.M. (1953): Convulsive effects of light stimulation in children. *Am. J. Dis. Child.* **86,** 170–183.

Bickford, R.G., Klass, D.W. (1969): Sensory precipitation and reflex mechanisms. In: Jasper H.H, Ward A.A, Pope A. (eds). *Basic mechanism of the epilepsies.* Boston Little Brown Co. pp. 543–564.

Brausch, C.C., Ferguson, J.H. (1965): Colour as a factor in light-sensitive epilepsy.' *Neurol.* **15,** 154–164.

Gastaut, H. (1982): A new type of epilepsy: Benign partial epilpesy of childhood with occipital spikes. *Clin. Electroencephalogr.* **13,** 13–22.

Gastaut, H. (1985): Benign epilepsy of childhood with occipital paroxysms. In:Epileptic syndromes in infancy, childhood and adolescence. Roger *et al.* (Ed) London: John Libbey pp. 159–70.

Green, J.B. (1966): Self-induced seizures: clinical and electroencephalographic studies. *Arch. Neurol.* **15,** 579–586.

Green, J.B. (1968): The electroretinogram and visually evoked response in photosensitive epilepsy. *Trans. Am. Neurol. Assoc.* **93,** 95–8.

Gumnit, R.J., Niedermeyer, E., Spreen, O. (1965): Seizure activity uniquely inhibited by patterned vision. *Arch. Neurol.* **13,** 363–368.

Herrick, C.E. & Harding, G.F.A. (1980): The effect of sodium valporate on the photosensitive visual evoked potential. In: Barber, ed. Evoked Potentials. *Lancaster MPT Press,* pp. 539–545.

Harding, G.F.A. & Dimitrakoudi, M. (1977): The visual evoked potential in photosensitive epilepsy. In: Desmedt, J.E. (ed) *Visual evoked potentials in man:* New Developments. Oxford: Clarendon Press pp. 509–513.

Harding, G.F.A., Jeavons, P.M. & Edson, A.S. (1994): *Video material and epilepsy. Epilepsia,* 35(b), 1208–16.

Harding, G.F.A. & Jeavons, P.M. (1994): *Photosensitive epilepsy,* London: MacKeith Press.

Jeavons, P.M., Harding, G.F.A. & Bower, B.D. (1966): Intermittent photic stimulation in photosensitive epilepsy. *J. Electroencephalogr. Clin. Neurophysiol.* **21,** 308.

Jeavons, P.M. & Harding, G.F.A. (1975): Photosensitive epilepsy. London: Heinemann Medical Books (Clinics in Developmental Medicine No. 56.)

Jeavons, P.M., Harding, G.F.A. & Edson, A.S. (1994): Prognosis of photosensitivity – a further report. *Epilepsia,* (in press).

Kooi, K.A. (1971): *Fundamentals of electroencephalography.* New York: Harper & Row.

Maheshwari, M.C. & Jeavons, P.M. (1975): The clinical significance of occipital spikes as a sole response to intermittent photic stimulation. *Electroencephalogr. Clin. Neurophysiol.* **39,** 93.

Melsen, S. (1959): The value of photic stimulation in the diagnosis of epilepsy. *J. Nerv. Ment. Dis.* **128,** 508–519.

Pallis, C. & Louis, S. (1961): Television-induced seizures. *Lancet* i 188–190.

Panayiotopoulos, C.P. (1974): Effectiveness of photic stimulation on various eye-states in photosensitive epilepsy. *J. Neurol. Sci.* **23,** 165.

Panayiotopoulos, C.P., (1979): Conversion of photosensitive to scotosensitive epilepsy. *Neurology* **29,** 1550–1554.

Panayiotopoulos, C.P., (1981): Inhibitory effect of central vision on occipital lobe seizures. *Neurology* **31,** 1331–1333.

Panayiotopoulos, C.P., (1989): Fixation-off sensitive epilepsies. In: Beaumanoir, A. Gastaut, H. & Naquet, R., (eds) Reflex seizures and reflex epilepsies. International Symposium on Reflex Seizures and Reflex Epilepsies, Geneva, June 1988. Geneva: Médicine & Hygiene pp. 203–217.

Pantelakis, S.N., Bower, B.D. & Jones, H.D. (1962): Convulsions and television viewing. *BMJ* ii, 633–638.

Storm van Leeuwen, W. & Bekkering, D.H. (1958): Some results obtained with the EEG spectrograph. *J. Electroencephalogr. Clin. Neurophysiol.* **10,** 563–570.

Troupin, A.S. (1966): Photic activation and experimental data concerning coloured stimuli. *Neurology* **16,** 269–276.

Eyelid Myoclonia with Absences, edited by J.S. Duncan and C.P. Panayiotopoulos
© 1996 John Libbey & Company Ltd, pp. 77–87.

Chapter 10

The differentiation of 'eye closure' from 'eyes-closed' EEG abnormalities and their relation to photo- and fixation-off sensitivity

J.S. Duncan and C.P. Panayiotopoulos

National Hospital for Neurology and Neurosurgery, London, WC1N 3BG, UK and Neurophysiology and Epilepsies, St Thomas' Hospital, London, SE1 7EH, UK

Eyes-open, eyes-closed and eye closure in normal subjects

It has been demonstrated from the early days of the EEG that the recorded brain activity is different when the eyes are opened from when they are closed (Berger, 1929; Adrian & Matthews, 1934). The alpha rhythm is activated with eyes closed and attenuated with eyes opened.

Cruikshank (1937) observed that the frequency of the alpha-rhythm as it recovers from being blocked by light stimulus is higher than the prestimulation frequency (if one uses as a measure of post-stimulation frequency the first five alpha waves which appear). This effect was more noticeable when the intensity of light was high and decreased with decreasing intensity.

It has also been reported (Durrup & Fessard, 1935) and shown by EEG spectrographic methods (Storm van Leeuwen and Bekkering, 1958; Storm van Leewen *et al.,* 1960) that in some people the alpha rhythm is of higher frequency immediately after closing the eyes.

Thus in normal subjects the EEG activity is different while the eyes are opened (eyes-opened state), closed (eyes-closed state) or immediately after closing of the eyes (eye closure state).

Similarly, there are certain epileptic conditions in which the EEG paroxysms are specifically or predominantly related to the above three conditions.

Photosensitive, scotosensitive and fixation-off sensitive (FOS) epilepsies are often evident in the resting EEG before any specific tests are carried out. Photosensitivity is mainly associated with eye closure abnormalities which are eliminated in darkness. Fixation-off sensitivity and scotosensitivity are associated with eyes-closed abnormalities which are activated by elimination of central vision and fixation (Panayiotopoulos, 1994).

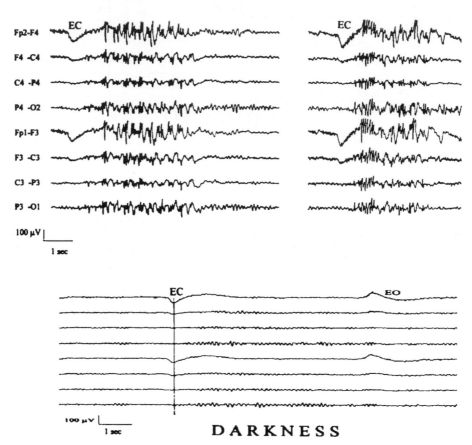

Fig. 1. *Eye closure (upper) abnormalities are induced immediately after closing of the eyes, are short and do not persist in the remaining period that the eyes are closed. They occur mainly in photosensitive patients and do not occur in darkness or probably in conditions of elimination of central vision and fixation.*
Upper: Video-EEG recording in a lit room in eyelid myoclonia with absences.
Lower: Eye-closure abnormalities are totally inhibited in conditions of complete darkness and elimination of central vision and fixation. (Modified from Giannakodimos & Panayiotopoulos, 1996 with the permission of the Editor of Epilepsia*).*

Thus, it is important to differentiate between *eye closure* (Fig. 1) and *eyes-closed* EEG (Figs. 2 and 3) abnormalities because of their different properties and their different response to light, darkness and elimination of central vision and fixation.

Eye closure abnormalities

Eye closure is the transient state which immediately follows the closing of the eyes. It lasts less than 3 s and does not persist for the remaining time during which the eyes are closed (Fig. 1). Eye closure induced abnormalities are mainly generalized, they occur within 2–4 seconds after closing of the eyes and are brief, usually lasting 1–4 seconds. Eye-closure transient EEG paroxysmal abnormalities occur mainly in photosensitive patients and are inhibited by darkness (Panayiotopoulos, 1972; 1974; 1977). The prevalence of eye closure discharges in photosensitive patients is 20 to 36

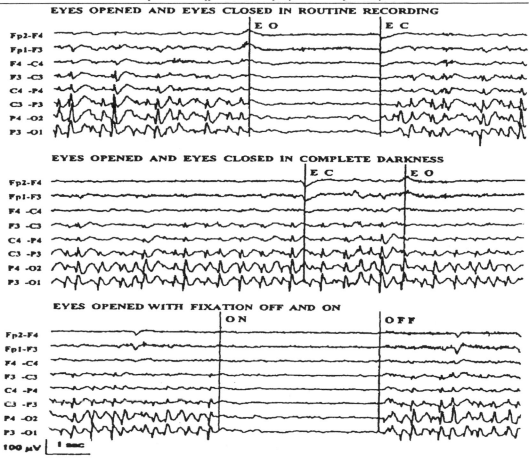

EYES OPENED AND EYES CLOSED IN ROUTINE RECORDING

EYES OPENED AND EYES CLOSED IN COMPLETE DARKNESS

EYES OPENED WITH FIXATION OFF AND ON

Fig. 2. Eyes-closed abnormalities and fixation-off sensitivity in an 11-year-old boy with late onset benign childhood epilepsy and occipital paroxysms (case 7 in Panayiotopoulos, 1993).
Upper: High amplitude sharp- and slow-wave occipital paroxysms are immediately induced after closing the eyes and persist as long as the eyes are closed (eyes-closed abnormalities) in a lit room. The results are identical whether fixation-off is achieved with closed eyelids, there is complete darkness, or +10 spherical lenses or underwater goggles covered with semitransparent tape are worn in the presence of light. Monocular fixation-off is not effective in eliciting occipital paroxysms irrespective of the method of eliminating central vision and fixation; similarly, occipital paroxysms are inhibited with binocular or monocular fixation. Middle: With elimination of central vision and fixation, inhibition does not occur with opening of the eyes. The occipital paroxysms become continuous irrespective of the eyes being closed or opened. Imaginary fixation (asking the patient to look at his/her thumb) during elimination of central vision does not inhibit the occipital paroxysms. Lower: Recording with eyes opened, excitation and inhibition are related not to eye opening and closing, but to fixation-on (with inhibition) and -off (with excitation).

per cent (Panayiotopoulos, 1972; Jeavons & Harding, 1975). The ideal model for the study of eye closure EEG abnormalities is eyelid myoclonia with absences (Panayiotopoulos, 1994; Gianna-kodimos & Panayiotopoulos, 1996).

Eyes-closed abnormalities

Eyes-closed is the state which persists as long as the eyes remain closed (Figs. 2 and 3). The eyes-closed abnormalities may be continuous or intermittent, generalized or focal, unilateral or

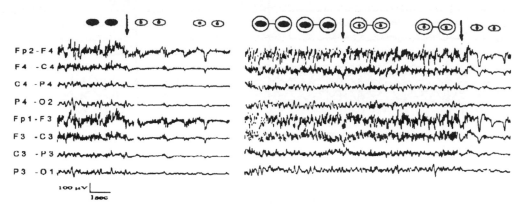

Fig. 3. Video-EEG recording in 1992 of a patient previously reported by Panayiotopoulos (1987a) with fixation-off sensitivity and intractable seizures.

EEG abnormalities and seizures occurred as soon as eyes were closed and were abruptly terminated on opening of the eyes in a lit room (right, symbols of eyes opened and eyes closed without glasses). However, eye opening was not effective in darkness and fixation-off was achieved by underwater goggles covered with opaque or semitransparent paper. In these conditions the paroxysomal activity continued irrespective of eyes closed or opened (left, symbols of eyes opened and eyes closed with glasses) and immediately stopped when fixation was allowed (extreme left). Darkness was quantitatively more effective than fixation-off in the presence of light (see text). Note that the alpha rhythm does not attenuate with eyes opened in darkness.

bilateral. The eyes-closed EEG abnormalities which are continuous and persist as long as the eyes remain closed are often activated by fixation-off sensitivity and scotosensitivity (Panayiotopoulos, 1981; 1987; 1989b; 1994).

Fixation-off sensitivity (FOS) refers to the forms of epilepsy and/or electroencephalographic (EEG) abnormalities which are elicited by elimination of central vision and fixation (Panayiotopoulos, 1981; 1987; 1989b; 1994).

FOS was first documented in children with the syndrome of benign childhood epilepsy with occipital paroxysms (Panayiotopoulos, 1981, 1987a; 1993) who have interictal EEG abnormalities which consist of continuous high amplitude occipital paroxysmal abnormalities as long as eyes are closed and which disappear for as long as the eyes are opened (Fig. 1).

It has been demonstrated that occipital paroxysms are activated by eyes-closed because of the elimination of central vision and fixation because they also occur when the eyes are opened providing the patient is deprived of central vision and fixation. Thus, with eyes opened the occipital paroxysms are immediately induced by complete darkness, vision through plus 10 spherical lenses or underwater goggles covered with semitransparent tape (in the presence of light). Under these circumstances of fixation-off, the occipital paroxysms are continuous and they are not reactive to eyes opened or closed (Fig. 2). The occipital paroxysms disappear again if central vision and fixation are restored either binocularly or monocularly (Fig. 2). In darkness the occipital paroxysms are totally inhibited by fixation on a small spot of low intensity red light (Panayiotopoulos, 1980; 1981).

Thus the occipital paroxysms are inhibited by fixation and activated by the absence of fixation even in the presence of light (Fig. 2).

Panayiotopoulos (1981; 1989b; 1994) concluded that the excitatory effect of darkness was in fact due to the elimination of central vision and fixation and that darkness was not a prerequisite for the activation of the occipital paroxysms. He coined the term 'fixation-off sensitivity' to distinguish it from scotosensitivity.

Fixation-off sensitivity has also been described in conditions other than of benign childhood epilepsy with occipital paroxysms. A case with atypical eyelid myoclonic absences, absence status and generalized tonic-clonic seizures who had eyes-closed but not eye closure induced clinical and EEG manifestations has been previously reported by Panayiotopoulos (1987).

This woman, born in 1954 and of borderline intelligence, had over the years many EEGs which showed generalized abnormalities of fast rhythms intermixed with spikes, multiple spikes and slow waves which were continuously recorded when her eyes were closed and abruptly terminated when the eyes were opened. The reactivity of these discharges to complete darkness and fixation on and off in the presence of light were identical to those described above for children with occipital paroxysms (Fig. 3). The only difference was that in darkness, total inhibition of the EEG abnormalities was achieved by a stronger light stimulus (a 2 cm spot of light of an ophthalmoscope projected on a white wall 3 m away from her eyes). Inhibition was not observed when a red spot of light was shown or the light of the ophthalmoscope was dimmed, although seen by the patient. Another interesting finding in this patient was that her alpha rhythm, on the few occasions that it could be seen, did not attenuate on eyes-opened in darkness. The same patient was recently re-evaluated with video-EEG (Panayiotopoulos, 1994). Once more, her EEG abnormalities and seizures were more marked and more consistent if the fixation point was intense or the environment darker. Clinically, her eyelids showed fast, small-range clonic movements associated with tonic spasm of the eyelids and eyes which were deviated upwards and laterally; the clonic movements occasionally spread to involve the neck muscles. These attacks were always related to eyes closed and the patient was not photosensitive.

Though initially this case was called 'eyelid myoclonia with absences', this diagnosis should strictly be reserved only for the syndrome described by Jeavons (1977), where all patients are photosensitive and show eye closure, not eyes-closed, abnormalities which are inhibited in darkness (Appleton *et al.,* 1993; Giannakodimos and Panayiotopoulos, 1996). The ictal clinical manifestations and the EEG abnormalities of the above patient are markedly different to those associated with the syndrome of 'eyelid myoclonia with absences' (Giannakodimos & Panayiotopoulos, 1996).

The case described by Gumnit *et al.* in 1965 had similar clinical and EEG manifestations to the above patient and is probably the first reported patient with FOS, although emphasis was given to the inhibitory effect of the patterned vision and not to fixation.

Another case reported by Barclay *et al.* (1993) may have had similar clinical and routine EEG manifestations to the above two patients. This was a 19 -year-old woman with mild mental retardation and intractable generalized seizures from the age 2 years. These were drop attacks, atypical absences, absence status and generalized tonic-clonic seizures. The EEG showed only, and as long as the eyes were closed, continuous high amplitude generalized beta activity which was superimposed on rhythmic delta activity and was associated with eyelid fluttering and impairment of cognition. This was not seen on eyes open, passive eye closure, use of Fenzel lenses or darkness. However, in darkness abnormalities initiated by eyes-closed were not attenuated by opening of the eyes but only after focusing on a red spot of light.

Similarly, many of the cases described as scotosensitive epilepsy (see below) may in fact be FOS.

Other types of EEG abnormalities and clinical manifestations may be found if FOS testing is introduced into EEG departments, as is the practice with intermittent photic stimulation and photosensitive epilepsy. The prevalence of FOS-related EEG abnormalities appears to be as frequent as that of photoconvulsive responses in children younger than 12 years of age (Panayiotopoulos, 1994).

Confirmation of fixation-off sensitivity

First, it is essential to confirm that the EEG abnormalities observed in routine EEG recording are eyes-closed related. The patient is asked to open and close his/her eyes every 5 seconds six times consecutively; ensure fixation in the eyes-opened state by instructing the patient to look at a fixed point (the tip of a pencil would do). Second, test for FOS by instructing the patient to perform the same sequence of eyes-opened and eyes-closed as above (six sequential trials of 5 seconds eyes-opened and eyes-closed) in conditions in which central vision and fixation are eliminated.

There are many ways to achieve this; a practical method is to ask the patient to wear a pair of underwater goggles which are fitted with +10 spherical lenses or semitransparent tape.

Elimination of central vision and fixation through total darkness is difficult to achieve in routine EEG departments because of the light indicators on equipment EEG and other machines as well as light coming through door and window openings; it should be remembered that FOS EEG abnormalities introduced in total darkness are dramatically inhibited when the patient fixates on a small red spot of light. It is our practice to test the effect of darkness with the patient wearing another pair of underwater goggles in which light has been totally blanked out with an opaque (non-transparent) tape.

Pitfalls in detecting eye closure and eyes-closed EEG abnormalities

To categorize the EEG abnormalities as eye closure or eyes-closed related, there should be an unequivocal relation to eye closure or eyes-closed. Spontaneous EEG paroxysmal abnormalities tend to increase on eye closure and eyes-closed. These cannot be studied properly without statistically adequate trials. There are many reports of the effect of darkness and proprioceptive impulses on EEG abnormalities which occur after closing of the eyes and disappear when the eyes are opened. There are many reasons for the apparently contradictory conclusions in some reports that darkness has no effect, in others inhibition, and in yet others activation:

(a) Paroxysmal abnormalities with eyes closed is often not distinguished from that with eye closure.

(b) The effect of darkness has often been studied either in a darkened room without elimination of central vision and fixation, or in 'total' darkness in which the patient may still be able to fixate on small light sources.

(c) Passively holding the eyes open while the patient forcibly tries to close them may eliminate fixation through Bell's phenomenon.

(d) It is not stated whether the trials in different conditions were sufficient to exclude a chance response particularly in patients with spontaneous EEG abnormalities.

(e) Patients, photosensitive or not, often had different epilepsy diseases or syndromes.

(f) EEG abnormalities were also often heterogeneous, varying from a brief generalized discharge, either consistently or occasionally induced or increased by eye closure, to recruiting responses, 3 Hz spike and slow waves of typical absences, and posterior or even unilateral spike and slow wave activity.

Illustrative review of the literature

Walter & Walter (1949) stated that in some patients intermittent photic stimulation is effective only at the moment of closing the eyes.

Atzev (1962) reported the effect of closing and opening the eyes upon the epileptic EEG activity. In 29 out of 1000 patients with epileptic seizures, EEG abnormalities in the form of spikes and sharp wave complexes were provoked by closing the eyes and in several patients absences were induced.

Jeavons (1966) reported that of 402 patients with photoparoxysmal EEG responses, 7 per cent showed spontaneous spike/polyspike and wave discharges immediately following the closing of the eyes (eye-closure related abnormalities).

Green (1968) reported four patients with *seizures on closing the eyes* which could also occur in darkness, although a diminishing effect was noted in one of them. The effect of fixation cannot be excluded in these. Three patients were photosensitive and at least one of them had eyelid myoclonia with absences. Patient 2, a 6 year old girl who was not photosensitive, had a single left sided convulsion. The EEG showed high amplitude spike and slow wave complexes predominantly on the right which were mainly induced by forceful closure of the eyes and sustained as long as this was maintained. Eye closure induced attacks even in darkness. This may be an example of seizures induced by proprioceptive stimuli from the ocular and/or eyelid muscles.

Panayiotopoulos (1972) found eye closure related abnormalities in 14 out of 70 patients with photoconvulsive responses. In six of them this was the only detectable abnormality in the resting EEG. More importantly, in five photosensitive patients brief generalized discharges consistently elicited by eye closure in an illuminated room were totally inhibited if eye closure was performed in complete darkness (Panayiotopoulos, 1972; 1974). Two of these patients also had alpha 'squeak' (a transitory increase of alpha activity amplitude and frequency after eye closure (Storm van Leeuwen *et al.*, 1960) in a well lit environment, which disappeared in darkness.

Lewis (1972) presented 2 patients with 'eye closure as a motor trigger for seizures'. Patient 1 was a 6 year old boy of borderline intelligence with intractable atypical absences, myoclonic jerks with massive flexion spasms, drop attacks and generalized tonic-clonic seizures. He also had multiple occipital spikes at 9–13 Hz which occurred within 1 s after closing of the eyes and persisted, "waxing and waning usually dying out gradually" while the eyes remained closed. These occipital discharges were clinically associated with rapid eyelid clonus and mild impairment of cognition. He was not photosensitive: 'virtually total darkness,' which may not have been complete, did not alter this pattern. Patient 2, a 13 year-old boy, had typical absence seizures and two generalized tonic-clonic seizures. The EEG during absences showed generalized multiple spikes followed by 3–4 Hz spike and multiple spike and slow wave activity. The absences were induced mainly on eye closure (55 per cent of eye closures induced seizures, including those in which the discharge did not occur immediately but after 10–16 seconds), intermittent photic stimulation and voluntarily squeezing the passively closed eyes. Darkness, possibly not complete, and squeezing the passively open eyes did not alter the above pattern.

Jeavons & Harding (1975) in their classic monograph on photosensitive epilepsy concluded that eye closure abnormalities were not usually present in darkness. They also reported a photosensitive patient with generalized discharges induced by changing the direction of gaze and another one who had polyspikes and myoclonic jerks on eye opening.

Vignaendra *et al.* (1976) reported two patients with 'epileptic discharges triggered by blinking and eye closure'. Patient 1 was a 10 year old of low intelligence with a history of persistent febrile convulsions. EEG showed that each blink elicited a high amplitude occipital sharp and slow wave complex which would appear in runs lasting as long as the eyes were closed. The sharp waves would also be induced by forced eye closure while the eyelids were held open. There was no difference in this pattern in darkness or light. There was no photosensitivity. They concluded that sensory afferents from the orbicularis oculi may have been the epileptic trigger. Patient 2 of Vignaendra *et al.* was a girl with marked photosensitivity and brief absences also induced by eye closure.

Klass (in Naquet, 1976) briefly described a patient who responded to pattern withdrawal, intermittent photic stimulation, eye closure and pattern stimulation with spike and wave discharges and concurrent myoclonus.

Darby *et al.* (1980) reported seven photosensitive patients with generalized spike and multiple spike and slow wave discharges following slow partial or complete eye closure of 1–2 seconds duration often with marked upward deviation of the eyes. None of these patients had discharges on voluntary eye closure except one who then performed a similar slow eye closure. The incidence of slow eye closure was reduced (four patients) or abolished (three patients) when room lighting was dimmed. Switching the lights off with the eyes open did not elicit any discharges. Five of these patients admitted to or had a history of self-induction.

Rafal et al. (1986) described a mentally retarded girl with Lennox-Gastaut syndrome who could induce seizures with eyeblinks in light and darkness; a blink could also be the only clinical manifestation, preceded by an EEG discharge. She was not photosensitive. 'The most effective activator of seizures was blinking triggered by social stress or cognitive effort.'

De Marco (1989) described identical twins who from age 4 had frequent absences characterized by 'palpebral flutter, loss of consciousness and upward deviation of the eyeball'. These were consistently induced by eye closure in light and darkness and not by intermittent photic stimulation.

Gobbi et al. (1989) found 51 published patients with epileptiform discharges elicited with eyes closed and/or eye closure. They reviewed 24 patients, of whom 16 were also photosensitive, and data were inadequate for the remaining 27. They also studied 22 patients with 'eye closure seizures', 11 of which had eyelid myoclonia with absences and photosensitivity. The remaining 11 patients fell into two groups:

(a) Five patients, three of whom were photosensitive, had predominantly or exclusively eye closure seizures which occurred within seconds of closing the eyes and did not persist through the eyes-closed period. The eye closure induced seizures consisted of bilateral myoclonic jerks or absences with myoclonia of 2–5 seconds, associated with generalized spike or multiple spike discharges.

(b) Six patients, four of whom were photosensitive, had repetitive myoclonic jerks induced by closing of the eyes and persisting as long as the eyes were closed. The EEG consisted of an initial rapid recruiting rhythm followed by multiple spike and wave discharges concomitant with the jerks.

The eye closure or eyes-closed related paroxysmal abnormalities in both groups appeared to persist in darkness and light though fixation may not have been excluded; their time of onset was not different in the four non-photosensitive patients but a delay in their appearance was noted in the seven photosensitive patients.

Imagaki et al. (1991) reported an infant with 'myoclonic astatic epilepsy'. He was not photosensitive but had eye closure induced myoclonic eyelid seizures in light and darkness. A Bell's phenomenon seemed necessary to trigger the seizures. Duncan et al. (1991) reported a woman with non-ketotic hyperglycaemia and gaze-evoked visual seizures which disappeared after correction of the hyperglycaemia. The seizures were consistently elicited within 2–3 seconds of looking to the left and consisted of hallucinations starting with a luminous ball in her left visual field, which was temporarily hemianopic, and concurrent rhythmic right temporo-occipital paroxysmal abnormalities. Partial motor seizures triggered by passive or voluntary movements, including those of the head and eyes, are well known in non-ketotic hyperglycaemia (see Duncan et al., 1991).

Other reports on eyes-closed and eye closure EEG abnormalities can be found in Pampiglione, 1951; Gastaut & Tassinari, 1966; Green, 1966; Giovanardi Rossi et al., 1969; Aguglia et al., 1985; Striano et al., 1979 ; De Marco & Miottello, 1981; Lugaresi et al., 1984; Cirignotta et al., 1987; Fabian & Wolf, 1987; Kohno et al., 1987; Newton & Aicardi, 1983, Beaumanoir et al., 1981; 1989).

Speculations on the generation of eye closure paroxysmal abnormalities in photosensitive patients

The underlying mechanisms for eliciting the eye closure paroxysmal abnormalities in photosensitive patients are not known and various speculations have been made:

(a) Activation of off-responding visual neurones (Panayiotopoulos, 1974). However, it is unlikely that a sudden reduction in retinal illumination is the mechanism responsible because switching the room lights off may not induce paroxysmal abnormalities (Darby et al., 1980) and in patients with eyelid myoclonia with absences, eye closure paroxysmal abnormalities persist despite remission of photosensitivity (Fabian & Wolf, 1987; Gobbi *et al.*, 1989; Panayiotopoulos, 1994).

(b) A flickering effect caused by oscillations of the eyeball and tremor of the eyelids when the eyes are voluntarily turned maximally upwards, thus inducing intermittent retinal stimulation (Darby *et al.*, 1980). This is also unlikely because of the persistence of eye closure abnormalities despite remission of photosensitivity.

(c) Voluntary eye closure may, as a result of repeated association with a visual stimulus that elicits paroxysmal abnormalities, condition the discharges to the proprioceptive feedback of eye closure (Darby *et al.*, 1980).

(d) Proprioceptive impulses generated by eye closure or the mechanisms associated with moving the eyes may trigger paroxysmal abnormalities (Green, 1968; Lewis, 1972). This cannot be true in patients whose eye closure discharges disappear in darkness.

(e) The paroxysmal abnormalities induced by eye closure may be related to a mechanism of alpha rhythm augmentation (Panayiotopoulos, 1972; Darby *et al.*, 1980). This is the strongest possibility because the alpha squeak phenomenon (see above) also appears to be eliminated in darkness (Panayiotopoulos, 1972; 1994), although more systematic studies are needed.

Acknowledgements

The Special Trustees of St.Thomas' Hospital are acknowledged for grants to CPP for his studies on epilepsies.

References

Adrian, E.D. & Matthews, B.H.C. (1934): The Berger rhythm: Potential changes from the occipital lobes in man. *Brain* **57,** 355–385.

Aguglia, U., Tinuper, P., Gobbi, G. & Gastaut, H. (1985): Absence status appearing on eye closure. *Clin. Electroencephalogr.* **16,** 111–118.

Appleton, R., Panayiotopoulos, C.P., Acomb, A.B. & Beirne, M. (1993): Eyelid myoclonia with absences: an epilepsy syndrome. *J. Neurol. Neurosurg. Psychiatry* **56,** 1312–1316.

Atzev, E. (1962). The effect of closing of the eyes upon epileptic activity of the brain. *Electroencephalogr. Clin. Neurophysiol.* **14,** 561.

Barclay, C.L., Murphy, W.F., Lee, M.A. & Zarwish, H.Z. (1993): Unusual form of seizures induced by eye closure. *Epilepsia* **34,** 289–290.

Beaumanoir, A., Capizzi, G., Nahori, A., and Yousfi, Y. (1989): Scotogenic seizures. In: *Reflex seizures and reflex epilepsies,* edited by A. Beaumanoir, H. Gastaut, and R. Naquet, pp. 219–223. Medecine & Hygiene, Geneva.

Beaumanoir, A., Inderwildi, B. & Zagury, S. (1981). Paroxysms EEG non epileptiques. *Med. Hyg.* **1425,** 1911–1918.

Berger, H. (1929): Uber das Elektrenkephalogramm des Menschen. *Arch. Psychiat. Nervenkr.* **87,** 527.

Cirignotta, F., Lugaresi, E. & Montana, P. (1987): Occipital–EEG activity induced by darkness: the critical role of central vision. In: *Migraine and epilepsy,* edited by F. Andermann and J. Lugaresi, pp. 139–143. New York: Raven Press.

Cruikshank, R.M. (1937): Human occipital brain potentials as affected by intensity-duration variables of visual stimulation. *J. Esp. Psychol.* **21,** 625–641.

Darby, C.E., De Court, R.A., Binnie, C.D. & Wilkins, A.J. (1980): The self-induction of epileptic seizures by eye-closure. *Epilepsia* **21,** 31–41.

De Marco, P. (1989): Eyelid myoclonia with absences in two monovular twins. *Clin. Electroencephalogr.* **20,** 193–195.

De Marco, P. & Miottello, P. (1981): Eye closure epilepsy, report of an uncomplicated case. *Clin. Electroencephalogr.* **12,** 66–68.

Duncan M.B., Jabbari, B. & Rosenberg, M.L (1991): Gaze-evoked visual seizures in nonketotic hyperglycaemia. *Epilepsia* **31,** 221–224.

Durrup, G. & Fessard, A. (1935): L'electroencephalogramme de l'homme: observations psycho-physiologique relatives à l'actions des stimuli visuel et auditif. *Ann. Psychol.* **35,** 1–35.

Fabian, A. & Wolf, P. (1987): Epileptic discharges after eye-closure: relation to photosensitivity. In: *Advances in Epileptology,* edited by P. Wolf *et al..,* pp. 259–264. New York: Raven Press.

Gastaut, H. & Tassinari, C.A. (1966): Triggering mechanisms in epilepsy. The electroclinical point of view. *Epilepsia* **7,** 85–138.

Giannakodimos, S. & Panayiotopoulos, C.P. (1996): Eyelid myoclonia with absences: a clinical and video-EEG study in adults. *Epilepsia* **37,** 36–44.

Giovanardi Rossi, P., Frank, L., & Pazzaglia, P. (1969): Crisi epilettiche alla chiusura degli occhi. *Giorn Psichiatr Neuropatol* **67,** 469–476.

Gobbi., G., Bruno., L., Mainetti., A., Parmegianni., A., Tullini., A., Salvi., F., Tassinari., C.A., Santanelli, P., Bureau, M., Dravet, C.H., & Roger, J. (1989): Eye-closure seizures. In: *Reflex seizures and reflex epilepsies,* edited by A. Beaumanoir, H. Gastaut & R. Naquet, pp. 181–191. Medecine et Hygiene, Geneva.

Green, J.B. (1966): Self-induced seizures: clinical and electroencephalographic studies. *Arch. Neurol.* **15,** 579–586.

Green, J.B. (1968): Seizures on closing the eyes: electroencephalographic studies. *Neurology* **18,** 391–396.

Gumnit, R.J., Niedermeyer, E. & Spreen, O. (1965): Seizure activity uniquely inhibited by patterned vision. *Arch. Neurol.* **13,** 363–368.

Imagaki. M., Suzuki, N., Koeda, T., Kamuro, K. & Ohtani, K. (1991): Myoclonic astatic epilepsy presenting eyelid myoclonic seizures induced by closing of the eyes. *Jpn. J. Psychiatry Neurol.* **45,** 455–457.

Jeavons, P.M. (1966): Summary of papers on abnormalities during photic stimulation. *Proc. Electrophysiol. Technol. Ass.* **13,** 153–157.

Jeavons, P.M. (1977): Nosological problems of myoclonic epilepsies in childhood and adolescence. *Dev. Med. Child. Neurol.* **19,** 3–8.

Jeavons, P.M., & Harding, G.F.A. (1975): *Photosensitive epilepsy.* (Clinics in Developmental Medicine) **56,** London: Heinemann.

Kohno, C., Terasaki, T., Matsuda, M., Ohtsuka, Y,, Yamatogi, Y., Oka, E. & Ohtahara, S. (1987): Epilepsies with seizure discharges induced by eye closure. *Arch. Epileptol.* **16,** 251–253.

Lewis, J.E. (1972): Eye closure as a motor trigger for seizures. *Neurology* **22,** 1145–1150.

Lugaresi, E., Cirignotta, F., & Montagna, P. (1984): Occipital lobe epilepsy with scotosensitive seizures. *Epilepsia* **25,** 115–120.

Naquet, R., editor (1976): Activation and provocation methods in clinical neurophysiology. In: *Handbook of electroencephalography and clinical neurophysiology,* edited by A. Ramond (editor-in-chief). Vol. 3, part D, pp. 17–25. Elsevier, Amsterdam.

Newton, R., & Aicardi, J. (1983): Clinical findings in children with occipital spike-wave complexes suppressed by eye-opening. *Neurology* **33,** 1526–1529.

Pampiglione, G. (1951). Scosse miocloniche pressoche continue soppresse da stimuli. *Riv. Neur.* **21,** 368.

Panayiotopoulos, C.P. (1972): A study of photosensitive epilepsy with particular reference to occipital spikes induced by intermittent photic stimulation. PhD Thesis, University of Aston in Birmingham

Panayiotopoulos, C.P. (1974): Effectiveness of photic stimulation on various eye states in photosensitive epilepsy. *J. Neurol. Sci.* **23,** 165--173.

Panayiotopoulos, C.P. (1977): 'Eye closure' and 'eyes closed' EEG abnormalities: discrimination and effectiveness of light and dark. *Electroencephalogr. Clin. Neurophysiol.* **43,** 523.

Panayiotopoulos, C.P. (1980): Basilar migraine? Seizures and severe epileptiform EEG abnormalities. *Neurology* **30,** 1122–1125.

Panayiotopoulos, C.P. (1981): Inhibitory effect of central vision on occipital lobe seizures. *Neurology* **31,** 1331–1333.

Panayiotopoulos, C.P.(1987): Fixation-off sensitive epilepsy in eyelid myoclonia with absence seizures. *Ann. Neurol.* **22,** 87–89.

Panayiotopoulos, C.P. (1989a): Benign childhood epilepsy with occipital paroxysms: a 15 year prospective study. *Ann. Neurol.* **26,** 51–56.

Panayiotopoulos, C.P. (1989b): Fixation-off-sensitive epilepsies. In: *Reflex seizures and reflex epilepsies*, edited by A. Beaumanoir, H. Gastaut & R. Naquet, pp. 203–217. Medecine & Hygiene, Geneva.

Panayiotopoulos, C.P. (1993): Benign childhood epilepsy with occipital paroxysms In: *Occipital seizures and epilepsies in children*, edited by F. Andermann, A. Beaumanoir, L. Mira, J. Roger & C.A. Tassinari, pp. 151–196. London: John Libbey.

Panayiotopoulos, C.P. (1994): Fixation-off sensitive epilepsies: clinical and EEG characteristics. In: *Epileptic seizures and syndromes,* edited by P. Wolf. pp. 55-66. London.: John Libbey.

Rafal, R.D., Laxer, K.D., Janowsky, J.S. (1986): Seizures triggered by blinking in a non-photosensitive epileptic. *J. Neurol. Neurosurg. Psychiatry* **49,** 445–447.

Shanzer, S., April, R., & Atkin, A. (1965): Seizures induced by eye deviation. *Arch. Neurol.* **13,** 621–625.

Storm van Leeuwen W., & Beckerring, I.D.H. (1958): Some results obtained with the EEG-spectrograph. *Electroencephalogr. Clin. Neurophysiol.* **10,** 563–570.

Storm van Leeuwen W., Kemp, A., Kniper, J. (1960): Concerning the 'Squeak' phenomenon of the alpha rhythm. *Electroencephalogr. Clin. Neurophysiol.* **12,** 244.

Striano, S., Fels, A., Vacca, G., and Cadorna, A.M. (1979): Epileptic seizures on closing the eyes and upon the sudden disappearance of light. *Acta Neurol. (Napoli)* **1, D** 443–451.

Vignaendra, V., Thiam, G., Loh, G.L., & Lim, S.T.C (1976):Epileptic discharges triggered by blinking and eye closure. *Electroencephalogr. Clin. Neurophysiol.* **40,** 491–498.

Walter, V.J. & Walter, W.G. (1949): The central effect of rhythmic sensory stimulation. *Electroencephal. Clin. Neurophysiol.* **1,** 57–86.

Eyelid Myoclonia with Absences, edited by J.S. Duncan and C.P. Panayiotopoulos
© 1996 John Libbey & Company Ltd, pp. 89–92.

Chapter 11

Differential diagnosis of eyelid myoclonia with absences and self-induction by eye closure

C.D. Binnie

Department of Clinical Neurophysiology, The Maudsley Hospital, Denmark Hill, London, SE5 8AZ

The first unequivocal account of photosensitive epilepsy appears to be that by Radovici *et al.* (1932) of a patient with self-induced seizures. The patient habitually turned his head towards the sun, made rapid movements with his eyelids, and eventually lost consciousness and fell (see Appendix to Chapter 12). A decade later, Walter & Dovey (1946) demonstrated that epileptiform EEG discharges can be elicited by intermittent photic stimulation in susceptible subjects, and the introduction by Cobb (1947) of this technique into routine clinical EEG practice led to the recognition of photosensitivity as a seizure precipitant in some 4 per cent of people with epilepsy.

Many photosensitive epileptic subjects use their photosensitivity to induce seizures or apparently sub-clinical epileptiform discharges. Despite Radovici's report, most early accounts describe patients, usually mentally handicapped, who produced flicker by waving the outspread fingers of one hand in front of the eyes whilst staring at a bright light (Andermann *et al.*, 1962). Others used linear patterns for self induction, or deliberately approached environmental sources of flicker such as television sets (Andermann, 1971).

However, Green (1966) described a series of nine photosensitive patients with self-induced seizures, an unspecified number of whom (at least four) employed eye closure as the inducing manoeuvre; he described four further patients in 1968. He described the movement variously as 'blinking', 'eye closure' or 'clonic jerking' of the eyelids. Some of his illustrations show bursts of EMG activity accompanying the movement; some show a slow sustained oculographic artifact indicating closure rather than blinking. Detailed descriptions of the inducing movements based on video EEG and electro-oculogram (EOG) recordings are given by Darby *et al.* (1980) and Binnie *et al.* (1980). The eye movement is readily mistaken for a nervous tic, or for eyelid flutter accompanying an absence seizure, particularly in known photosensitive patients and those who may have eyelid myoclonia with absences (EMA). However, the eye closure itself is generally slow and sustained with greater than usual upward deflection of the globe, producing an EOG deflection clearly different from that of spontaneous blinking or eye-closure to command, neither of which produce the characteristic discharges in these patients. A tremor of the eyelids at about 6 Hz may be superimposed upon the eye closure. Whereas most patients using the very conspicuous manoeuvre of hand-waving are mentally handicapped, many of those using eye closure are of normal intelligence. Combined EEG telemetry and video monitoring of substantial series of photosensitive subjects suggests that some 24–37 per cent (Darby *et al.*, 1980; Binnie *et al.*, 1980; Kasteleijn-Nolst Trenité, 1989) engage in self-induction when placed in a well-lit environment, particularly if stressed.

Diagnostic criteria

Diagnostic features which may help to distinguish the phenomenon from involuntary ictal eyelid myoclonia are:

(1) the eye movement precedes the epileptiform EEG discharge;

(2) the oculographic artefact is larger and slower than that accompanying normal spontaneous eye closure and often shows a superimposed ocular tremor at about 6 Hz;

(3) the manoeuvre continues to be carried out, initially at least, when the patient is placed in darkness or when one eye is covered, but fails to produce an epileptiform discharge;

(4) when the environment is darkened or one eye covered there is a gradual extinction of the behaviour, so that the movements occurring without discharges are produced less frequently;

(5) the behaviour is increased by stress (reported by 12/37 of patients in the series of Kastelijn-Nolst Trenité, 1989), and occurs during inactivity with apparent boredom during prolonged recordings;

(6) most patients either have learning difficulties or show some degree of psychiatric abnormality;

(7) patients display guilt when the phenomenon is discussed;

(8) patients admit to carrying out the manoeuvre, variously describing it as voluntary or compulsive;

(9) a pleasant sensation is often reported; this may have a sexual component leading to orgasm in some subjects;

(10) there may be a history of seizures induced by hand-waving in the past or patients may use hand-waving in combination with slow eye closure to enhance or prolong the discharge, as documented on film by Ames (1974);

(11) this behaviour can usually be abolished by dopamine antagonists.

Of the above, perhaps the most compelling evidence of self-induction, as opposed to spontaneous eyelid myoclonia with absences, is the testimony of the patients themselves. In the largest reported series, derived from unselected referrals of people with epilepsy to an EEG service (Kastelijn-Nolst Trenité, 1989), 29 out of 100 photosensitive subjects admitted to self-induction; all but one used the eye closure manoeuvre. As sensations are reported or presumed to accompany the discharges, these are not strictly subclinical even if no seizure is observed. However, overt ictal events are often present, ranging from typical absences or myoclonic seizures to tonic-clonic convulsions.

Treatment

Self-induction of seizures is often resistant to therapy, not least because of non-compliance on the part of the subject (Andermann *et al.*, 1962; Rail, 1971; Kastelijn-Nolst Trenité *et al.*, 1989). Self-induction appears to be increased in stressful situations and is reported by some subjects as relieving anxiety; psychotherapy has proved effective (Libo *et al.*, 1971). Self-induction may be controlled with dark glasses in those patients who can be persuaded to wear them. Antiepileptic drugs are rarely effective but dopamine antagonists block self-induction. The rationale of this treatment is the observation that electrical self-stimulation of mesial brainstem structures in experimental animals is suppressed by these drugs (Olds *et al.*, 1956). Presumably dopamine antagonists, although proconvulsive and known to increase photosensitivity (Quesney *et al.*, 1980; Quesney, 1981) suppress self-induction by reducing the rewarding effect of the discharges (Kasteleijn-Nolst Trenité *et al.*, 1989). In two trials (Overweg & Binnie, 1980; Kastelijn-Nolst Trenité *et al.*, 1989) 12 out of 15 patients showed a reduction in self-induction (quantified by telemetric monitoring), but few were willing to accept long term treatment, as they had little interest in being relieved of their symptoms.

Eyelid myoclonias with absences

The account above of self-induction by eye closure is closely similar to the description by Jeavons (1977) of 'eyelid' myoclonia with 'absences': myoclonic jerks of the eyelids on eye closure in a photosensitive patient, accompanied by very fast spike-wave discharges. A more common finding, however, is of spike-wave activity on eye closure in a photosensitive subject, without overt clinical change (Crighel, 1963).

Whether eyelid myoclonia with absences forms a single discrete entity is debatable. Gobbi *et al*, (1989) provide a review of the literature, report 22 personal cases of seizures on eye closure and distinguish two subgroups. Some patients (group A) had brief myoclonias and absences and often other, spontaneous seizures. Others (group B) had continuing myoclonus with closed eyes generally without spontaneous seizures; their attacks were not strictly absence seizures. Photosensitivity was reported in most, but not in all patients, of both groups. It may appear before the development of eye-closure seizures, or disappear while these are still present. Eye closure results in seizures, even when the patient is in darkness. However, the latency from closure to discharge is increased in darkness in the photosensitive subjects but not in the others. It appears that the trigger mechanisms in these patients are complex, and they probably do not form a homogeneous group, and suffer from various idiopathic syndromes, notably juvenile myoclonic epilepsy.

Conclusion

Behaviourally, self-induction and eyelid myoclonia may be indistinguishable, and indeed the syndromes may coexist. Absences with eyelid myoclonia may be self-induced. Conversely the movements used for self-induction may include a voluntary eyelid flutter even when the attempt at induction is unsuccessful. This latter situation can be identified when the movement occurs without any EEG discharge; when there is a discharge, it may be impossible to tell whether the eyelid flutter is voluntary or ictal.

From a practical clinical standpoint, it is important to identify self-induction as this has consequences for treatment and prognosis. If a photosensitive patient shows eyelid flutter on eye closure, both eyelid myoclonia with absences and self-induction should be considered. Specifically, before a diagnosis of eyelid myoclonia with absences is taken at face value and the attacks assumed to be involuntary, history taking and investigations should be addressed to determining whether or not the features of self-induction set out above are present.

References

Ames, F.R. (1974): Cinefilm and EEG recording during 'handwaving' attacks of an epileptic, photosensitive child. *Electroencephalogr. Clin. Neurophysiol.* **37**, 301–304.

Andermann, F. (1971): Self-induced television epilepsy. *Epilepsia* **12**, 269.

Andermann, K., Oaks, G., Berman, S., Cooke, P.M., Dickson, J., Gastaut, H., Kennedy, A., Margerison, J.H., Pond, D.A. & Tizard, J.P. (1962): Self-induced epilepsy. *Arch. Neurol.* **6**, 49–79.

Binnie, C.D., Darby, C.E., De Korte, R.A. & Wilkins, A.J. (1980) Self- induction of epileptic seizures by eyeclosure: incidence and recognition. *J. Neurol. Neurosurg. Psychiatry* **43**, 386–389.

Cobb, S. (1947): Photic driving as a cause of clinical seizures in epileptic patients. *Arch. Neurol. Psychiatry* **58**, 70–71.

Crighel, E. (1963): The EEG activating phenomena on closing the eyes. *Electroencephalogr. Clin. Neurophysiol.* **15,** 531.

Darby, C.E., De Korte, R.A., Binnie, C.D. & Wilkins, A.J. (1980): The self-induction of epileptic seizures by eye closure. *Epilepsia* **21,** 31–42.

Gobbi, G., Bruno, L., Mainetti, A., *et al.* (1989) Seizures induced by eye closure. In: Reflex seizures and reflex epilepsies, eds. A. Beaumanoir, H. Gastaut & R. Naquet, pp. 181–192. Geneva: Editions Médecine et Hygiène.

Green, J.B. (1966): Self-induced seizures: clinical and electroencephalographic studies. *Arch. Neurol.* **15,** 579–586.

Green, J.B. (1968): Seizures on closing the eyes: electrographic studies. *Neurology* **18,** 391–396.

Jeavons, P.M. (1977): Nosological problems of myoclonic epilepsies of childhood and adolescence. *Devel. Med. Child. Neurol.* **19,** 38.

Kasteleijn-Nolst Trenité, D.G.A. (1989): Photosensitivity in epilepsy: electrophysiological and clinical correlates. *Acta Neurol. Scand.* (Suppl. 125).

Kasteleijn-Nolst Trenité, D.G.A., Binnie, C.D., Overweg, J., Oosting, J. & Van Emde Boas, W. (1989): Treatment of self-induction in epileptic patients. In: *Reflex Seizures and Reflex Epilepsies,* eds. A. Beaumanoir, H. Gastaut & R. Naquet, pp. 439–445. Geneva: Editions Médecine & Hygiène.

Libo, S.S., Palmer, C. & Archibald, D. (1971): Family group therapy for children with self-induced seizures. *Am. J. Orthopsychiatry* **41,** 506–508.

Olds, J., Killam, K.F. & Bach-Y-Rita, P. (1956) Self-stimulation of the brain used as a screening method for tranquilizing drugs. *Science* **124,** 265–266.

Overweg, J. & Binnie, C.D. (1980): Pharmacotherapy of self-induced seizures. *Acta Neurol. Scand.* (Suppl.) **79,** 98.

Quesney, L.F. (1981): Dopamine and generalized photosensitive epilepsy. In: *Neurotransmitters, Seizures, and Epilepsy,* eds., P.L. Morselli, W. Loscher, K.G. Lloyd, B. Meldrum & B Chir, pp. 263–274. New York: Raven Press.

Quesney, L.F., Andermann, F., Lal, S. & Prelevic, S. (1980): Transient abolition of generalized photosensitive epileptic discharge in humans by apomorphine, a dopamine-receptor agonist. *Neurology* **30,** 1169–1174.

Radovici, A., Misirliou, V. & Gluckman, M. (1932): Epilepsie réflexe provoquée par excitations optiques des rayons solaires. *Rev. Neurol.* **1,** 1305–1308.

Rail, L.R. (1971): The treatment of self-induced photic epilepsy. *Proc. Aust. Ass. Neurol.* **9,** 121–123.

Walter, W. & Dovey, V.J. (1946): Analysis of the electrical response of the human cortex to photic stimulation. *Nature* **158,** 540–541.

Eyelid Myoclonia with Absences, edited by J.S. Duncan and C.P. Panayiotopoulos
© 1996 John Libbey & Company Ltd, pp. 93–106.

Chapter 12

Eyelid myoclonia is not a manoeuvre for self-induced seizures in eyelid myoclonia with absences

C.P. Panayiotopoulos, S. Giannakodimos, A. Agathonikou and
M. Koutroumanidis

Department of Clinical Neurophysiology and Epilepsies, St. Thomas' Hospital, London

Some reports and most epileptologists consider eyelid myoclonia with absences (EMA) to be a manoeuvre used by patients to self-induce intermittent photic stimulation and elicit seizures. Binnie & Jeavons (1992) suggested that the majority of patients with EMA suffer from self-induced seizures and that eyelid myoclonia is a self-induced manoeuvre. This does not appear to be correct. Neither Jeavons in his initial report (1977) nor ourselves (Appleton *et al.*, 1993: Giannakodimos & Panayiotopoulos, 1996; Panayiotopoulos, 1996b) considered eyelid myoclonia to be a manoeuvre employed by the patients for self-induction.

Our thesis, based on long video-EEG studies and extensive interviews with 15 adult patients with EMA, is that eyelid myoclonia is an epileptic seizure, an ictal manifestation, and not an attempt by the patient to self-induce intermittent light stimulation for the provocation of seizures. In patients with EMA, a normal light reflex eye closure or spontaneous eye blinks may elicit seizures manifested by eyelid myoclonia, often associated with jerks of the eyes and the head. This is not an attempt at self-induction. In patients with EMA, closing of the eyes (there is no need for forceful slow eye closure) in the presence of uninterrupted light may be more powerful than intermittent photic stimulation for the provocation of a seizure. Therefore, these patients do not need intermittent photic stimulation to induce seizures. Furthermore, some adult patients with EMA continue with eyelid myoclonia although minimum or no photosensitivity is manifested during intermittent photic stimulation (Giannakodimos & Panayiotopoulos, 1996; see also Chapter 8).

Self-induced seizures in photosensitive patients

Self-induced seizures in photosensitive patients are well known and well documented in the literature (Andermann *et al.*, 1962; Chao, 1962; Green, 1966; Ames; 1971; 1974; Panayiotopoulos, 1972; 1995; Tassinari *et al.*, 1989; 1990; Antebi & Bird 1993: Aicardi, 1994; Harding & Jeavons, 1994; Panayiotopoulos *et al.*, 1975; Duncan & Panayiotopoulos, 1995; Chapter 8). The best known

Self-induction in Photosensitive Epilepsy

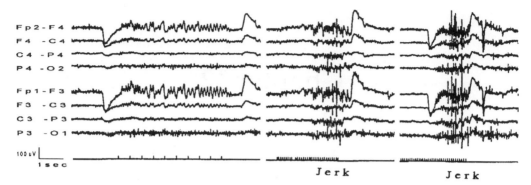

Fig. 1. Video-EEG of case 1 during intermittent photic stimulation.
Left: Voluntary eyelid fluttering without EEG abnormalities at low flash rates. Center and right:
Photoconvulsive discharges of polyspikes are induced by higher flash rates and these are clinically
manifested with axial and limb jerks. There was no eyelid myoclonia.

manoeuvre for self-induction is looking at a bright light source, usually the sun, and voluntarily waving the abducted fingers in front of the eyes ('sunflower syndrome'; Ames & Saffer, 1983) in order to induce intermittent photic stimulation. Other patients achieve intermittent photic stimulation and self-induced seizures with lateral or vertical rhythmic movements of the head, television and more recently video-games (Ferrie *et al.*, 1994).

It has also been well documented that some photosensitive patients may also have self-induced seizures by repetitive opening and closing of the eyes in front of a bright light source. These patients are simply photosensitive patients imitating EMA. We have seen such a patient and have recorded with video-EEG spontaneous and on–command eyelid myoclonia-like repetitive opening and closing of the eyelids (Fig. 1).

Case 1

Case 1 is a female, 22 years old. Onset of EMA-like eyelid blinking occurred at age 10-11 years. She is strongly and compulsively attracted to lights (mainly sun and fluorescent lights) where she manifests fast repetitive eye opening and closing. This is followed by axial and limb jerks and on three occasions generalized tonic-lonic seizures. She likes it, it relieves tension. 'I do not do it on purpose but I do not exactly avoid it ... I do not actually deliberately go out to find some bright light but if I find it I am happy ... I would like to stop doing it, but it is a funny nice feeling. I cannot say it is nice, it is a relief ... In a way, it is a play between me and the sun ... It is a mixture of feelings. On one hand I do not want to do it, but on the other hand it is releasing something ... No, it is not sexual ... I know it is strange.'

There is a strong family history of photosensitivity. Her brother is also photosensitive without evidence of self-induction. The maternal twin sister 'had many seizures, was after the lights and died at age 16 years during an epileptic attack'.

Video-EEG demonstrates spontaneous EMA-like symptoms which she can also imitate at request without EEG discharges. There are no abnormalities on eye closure and the photoconvulsive discharges are unlike those of EMA (Fig 1).

Other patients may have self-induced pattern sensitive epilepsy (Panayiotopoulos, 1979) and we have recently seen a photosensitive patient with absence seizures who confessed self-inducing seizures by stressful thinking (Fig. 2).

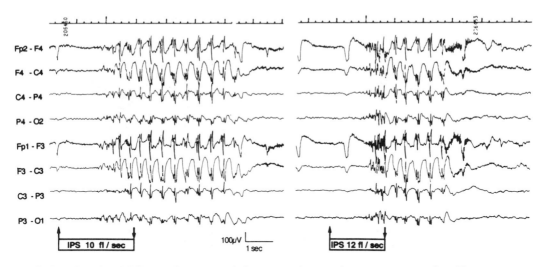

Fig. 2. Case 2. Video-EEG recording. Typical absences without ictal eye movements induced by intermittent photic stimulation. Patient is unresponsive and stares.

Case 2

Case 2 is a normal male, age 20 years. He started having typical absences and occasional generalized tonic-clonic seizures from childhood. Seizures occurred mainly after awakening or provoked by television and flickering lights. He was self-inducing seizures only by thinking:

"My epilepsy started a few months after my father died. I know when I self-induce the seizures. I could self-induce the seizures quite easily, if I thought about my father. Like the time that I spent with him, also the time that he was in the hospital or things like these. This could induce the seizures. I never did it to gain anything, I did it to get away from other people."

We are also aware of patients with EMA and self-induced seizures. We have reported in this book a girl with a family history of EMA who probably attempts to induce seizures with rapid horizontal movements of the head or hand waving (Chapters 6 & 12). Her mother had video-EEG documented eyelid myoclonia. She refused self-induction. The maternal identical twin sister also has eyelid myoclonia with persistent 'sunflower' movements of the fingers.

Slow eye closure and self-induction

Slow eye closure as a manoeuvre for self-induced seizures in photosensitive patients has been detailed by Binnie (see Chapter 10). Binnie *et al.*, (1980) described 13 patients who 'made repeated slow eye closure movements with simultaneous upward deviation of the eyes, considerably more marked than that ordinarily seen as the eyes are shut. Under conditions of normal room lighting this was usually followed by spike and wave or multiple spike and wave activity, either generalized or confined to the posterior regions of the head. In 11 patients one or more of these discharges was accompanied by a seizure, usually an absence. 'No patient volunteered a history of self-induction but eight admitted to the habit on direct questioning.'

There are many features in these patients which are unlike EMA. Only one of the patients had discharges elicited by eye closure to command. In their illustration slow eye closure elicited a generalized 3 Hz spike and slow wave of approximately 9 s duration which shows no similarities to the brief mainly multiple spike discharges of EMA. Two patients had partial seizures.

In another similar report by the same authors (Darby *et al.*, 1980), seven photosensitive patients

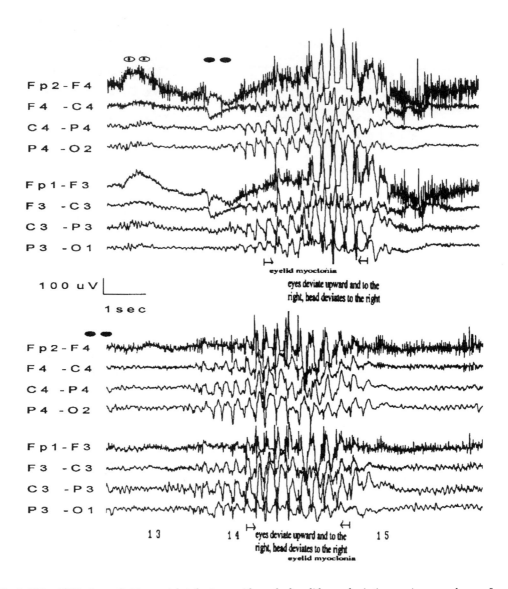

Fig. 3. Video-EEG of case 3. Upper: A brief seizure with marked eyelid myoclonia (arrows) on eye closure. Lower: A similar clinico-EEG seizure occurred while the eyes were closed and the patient was performing overbreathing with counting (numbers annotated). Eyelid myoclonia started well after the onset of the EEG discharge.

had generalized spike/multiple and slow discharges on EEG following partial or complete eye closure of 1–2 seconds duration (slow eye closure) often with marked upward deviation of the eyes. In none of the patients were such discharges recorded on voluntary eye closure to command except in one who was performing a similar slow eye closure. The incidence of slow eye closure was reduced (four cases) or abolished (three cases) when room lighting was dimmed. Switching the lights off with eyes open was not eliciting any discharges. Five of these patients admitted or had a history of self-induction. It is apparent from the illustrations that EEG discharges in some patients appeared before the completion of slow eye closure.

The same group of investigators (Wastell *et al.*, 1982) reported that a transient rise in EEG power at low frequencies 12 seconds before the eye closure was associated with the subsequent occurrence of paroxysmal activity. This was not seen before other slow eye closures or blinks not associated with paroxysmal activity. They speculated that this may reflect the launching of a contingent negative variation type of potential shift similar to those observed in preparation for action.

However, early forced eyelid blinking and flutter, myoclonic jerks of the eyelids and oculoclonic activity may be ictal manifestations of the occipital lobe seizures as documented with deep stereo-EEG recordings which may not show in surface EEG (Bancaud, 1969; Takeda *et al.*, 1970; Munari *et al.*, 1984; Williamson *et al.*, 1992).

In our experience with EMA, slow eye closure may occur but this is not a manoeuvre for self-induction as it often occurred at the end of a discharge or in between numerous clusters of eyelid myoclonia seizures, particularly on awakening. Also, it is difficult to explain slow eye closure as a manoeuvre for self-induction in EMA as we do not have any evidence that slow speed and force of closing of the eyes potentiates the EEG discharges.

Rafal *et al.* (1986) described a mentally retarded girl with Lennox-Gastaut syndrome who could induce seizures with eyeblinks in light and darkness but also in whom a blink could be the only clinical manifestation preceded by an EEG discharge. She was not photosensitive. 'The most effective activator of seizures was blinking triggered by social stress or cognitive effort'. The authors rightly, in our opinion, did not consider this as another case of self-induced epilepsy: 'her seizure activity behaviour did not appear to be willful or consciously generated'. They considered her to be of interest, to study the relationship between stress and seizure generation in view of the fact that 'blinking also functions as a complex indicator of phasic responses to stress such as that produced by listening to emotionally laden words' (Asher & Ort, 1951).

A 14 month old girl was reported as having self-induced seizures by blinking in front of the television. The evidence of self-induction was based on video-EEG recordings showing that the repetitive blinks occurred without EEG discharges which followed this behaviour. 'She learned to increase the brightness of the television picture....but IPS did not evoke paroxysmal discharges, probably because of the lack of patient's cooperation'(Watanabe *et al.*, 1985).

The same authors (Watanabe *et al.*, 1985) also reported a 2 year old boy as an example of self-induced photosensitive epilepsy. He had febrile and non-febrile generalized convulsions in the first year of his life. From the age of 12 months he started having frequent episodes in which he moved his head up while grimacing with the eyes half-closed (not associated with EEG changes. This was followed by motion arrest with staring or eyelid myoclonus and head drop which was associated with generalized spike and wave discharges. 'The head nodding behaviour ceased at the age of 3 years but he began to have myoclonic jerks induced by eyelid blinking.'

Whether these children at the age of 1 year can wilfully or consciously generate such a behaviour of self-induction may be open to debate.

EMA and the myth of self-induced seizures

The problem with EMA is that some investigators erroneously consider that the eyelid myoclonia is a self-induced attempt to induce intermittent photic stimulation and seizures. This belief is so strong that in nearly all relevant publications of self-induced seizures, the patient described by Radovici *et al.* (1932) is erroneously cited as the first reported case of self-induced seizures. No such evidence or mention of self-induced seizures can be found in reading the original report. On the contrary:

'AA ... age de 20 ans, présente des troubles moteurs sous forme de mouvements involontaires de la tête et des yeux sous l'influence des rayons solaires'.

As this is probably the first reported case of EMA and also the first case of experimental provocation of seizures documented with cine film it was decided to include in this book a complete translation of this paper in English (see Appendix).

Another widely cited paper on self-induced seizures is by Robertson (1954). He described seven patients with 'self-precipitated' attacks. Four of these waved their fingers in front of their faces. In the other three patients (two probably had EMA and the third had symptomatic eyelid myoclonia) it was presumed that 'flicker was produced by interrupting the sun's rays by blinking'. It is of note, however, that none of these patients had admitted self-induction. Case 7 was considered as self-induced eyelid myoclonia based on the following:

'the sun seems to do something to make me to look at it ... I do not know ... It does not give me any pleasure ... I cannot help it in one way, but when I think to stop it I stop ... I do not go out and sit in the sun ... '.

Robertson (1954) also described another case of EMA as a self-induced photosensitive epilepsy. This was the mother of a medical practitioner. 'Whenever she went into the sunlight her head went back and she blinked. A fleeting blankness of expression was recognisable. In addition she had suffered from 3 major convulsions 20, 17 and 2 years ago. These occurred after periods of overwork and stress'. Overwork and stress are well known precipitants of generalized tonic-clonic seizures in idiopathic generalized epilepsies and EMA. They should not be taken as evidence of self-induction.

A typical case of EMA often misinterpreted as a manoeuvre for self-induction

In our own experience, the best case to demonstrate EMA with home-made video is a 35 year old woman who had at least three ictal episodes of eyelid myoclonia during her wedding.

Case 3

Born in 1950, she is a successful sales manager. At age 4 years she developed frequent absences which were brief (4–7 s) associated with moderate impairment of cognition and marked eyelid myoclonia.

Absences improved but continued daily with ethosuximide. She became seizure-free when valproate was added to ethosuximide at age 31 years. Carbamazepine resulted in severe deterioration with eyelid myoclonia absence status and generalized tonic-clonic seizures.

She had a total of six generalized tonic-clonic seizures in her life, two induced by lights and the others after sleep deprivation, alcohol indulgence and inappropriate change of her medication.

Video-EEG studies demonstrated eyelid myoclonia with absences mainly on eye-closure and intermittent photic stimulation. Continuous clusters of eyelid myoclonia with and without absences occurred on awakening (see Fig. 1 in Giannakodimos & Panayiotopoulos, 1996).

When she was asked about the eyelid manifestations of her seizures, she said that she knew about them from descriptions of friends and that she had seen them in her wedding video. The most striking eyelid myoclonic seizures occurred as she was getting out of the car into the sun light to go to the church or posing for the wedding photographs in the sun. These episode of marked eyelid myoclonia induced by the sun are always considered by experienced audiences of epileptologists to whom this video is shown as a characteristic manoeuvre for self-induced seizures.

We argue that it is not:

(a) We have interviewed the patient many times and have performed four long video-EEGs during alert, sleep stages and awakening. We never had any evidence or suspicion that she had self-induced seizures. On the contrary, she was relieved when these seizures were controlled with the appropriate treatment which in her case was sodium valproate.

(b) Identical seizures, studied with video-EEG recordings, were elicited with intermittent photic stimulation, eye closure and also when the eyes were closed under circumstances of sleep deprivation on awakening. The seizures of eyelid myoclonia were simultaneous with generalized discharges of multiple spikes and slow waves; the latter could also precede the clinical manifestations (Fig. 3).

(c) Slow eye closure was seen only in the recording on awakening after partial sleep deprivation, when she was nearly in an eyelid myoclonia status.

The same patient had once a jerk of the head and on a few occasions mild eyelid myoclonia without EEG accompaniments. Should this be taken as evidence of self-induction? There is no reason to support such a proposal.

Results from a study of 17 adult patients with EMA

Clinical aspects

In interviews with 17 adult patients with EMA (Chapter 8), none of 15 patients admitted or was suspected of showing self-induced seizures. On the contrary, they considered eyelid myoclonia as a socially embarrassing condition and were relieved when the seizures improved. Furthermore, we consider it unlikely that self-induction would be attempted in the kinds of social situations we found by reviewing home videotapes.

> *'I will be looking over there and the sunshine will be coming through on that side. And my head, without me even knowing, it automatically turns, you cannot stop it and it goes like this and your head has an automatic reaction to go back to the sunlight and start flickering the eyes and you try to pull yourself away ... '*

This description may be arbitrarily taken as an indirect evidence of self-induction despite that this is strongly denied by the patients. To us, this is similar to the well known phenomenon of the 'attraction movement' when light is presented and other manifestations of the optic fixation reflexes when volitional movements of the eyes are unattainable or week (see for review Walsh, 1957).

Additionally, all 14 patients were anxious to receive medication and showed excellent compliance. In most of them eyelid myoclonia continued, although other types of seizures have been controlled. However, eyelid myoclonia was less severe and less frequent than before appropriate treatment. This is against self-induction where one would expect that eyelid myoclonia would be more forceful after treatment in order to induce seizures.

Two of the 17 patients were suspected of self-induction. One of them had frequent slow eye closure EEG abnormalities but she never admitted self-induction, and she takes her medication which has allowed her to obtain her driving license. She insisted, 'I do not know when I am doing it...It gives me no pleasure and it is a social embarrassment'. The other patient admitted in a video recorded interview that she occasionally does it voluntarily:

> *'Yes, I can do it on purpose like that (she imitates rapid eyelid blinking with upwards deviation of the eyes). But that is because there are times that my eyes start to want to go and do it and I know, they want to do it because they are strained and sore and they will sting and so if I just do it, it relaxes them ... That is a rare occasion. But other than that I do not know. It just goes on. There have been incidences I have walked into a pole, or into a car. I did not do that on purpose'.*

Video-EEG aspects

Sixteen of the 17 patients had abnormal video-EEG. All these 16 patients had eyelid myoclonia associated with EEG discharges which preceded or were simultaneously recorded with the eyelid symptoms. Eyelid myoclonia elicited while eyes were closed or opened was identical to that induced by closing of the eyes, and the associated EEG discharges were either simultaneous or preceded the clinical eyelid manifestations.

One patient with normal video-EEG had eyelid myoclonia with absences exacerbated by progesterone (Grunewald *et al.*, 1992).

Photosensitivity, which is a prerequisite for self-induction performed either by hand waving or eye blinking, was minimal (grade 1) in four of our patients with marked eyelid myoclonia on eye closure.

However, five patients also had video-EEG recorded episodes of eyelid myoclonia without EEG discharges but two of them also had axial or limb myoclonic jerks without EEG accompaniments. Also, most of the patients manifested with episodes of mild eyelid symptoms without EEG abnormalities. How may these be explained?

(a) *Attempts for self-induction.* Why? Eye closure could be more efficient at inducing seizures than photosensitivity which was minimal in some of these patients.

(b) *Seizures without EEG manifestations.* Possible, but difficult also to explain in view of the severe interictal EEG manifestations occurring in their EEGs. However, we have seen a young untreated girl with severe eyelid myoclonia and absences on eye closure who had a seizure of EMA associated with EEG discharges at onset but not in the subsequent 3 s of the clinical manifestations (see Fig. 3 of Chapter 3). She was not sensitive to intermittent photic stimulation. Furthermore, occipital lobe seizures may be manifested with eyelid jerks or blinks without scalp EEG changes (Bancaud, 1969; Takeda *et al.*, 1970; Munari *et al.*, 1984; Williamson *et al.*, 1992).

(c) *Conditioning.* This is likely but highly speculative (Darby *et al.* 1980).

(d) *Exaggeration of eyelid emotionally-related spontaneous movements seen in normal adult populations.* Why not?

(e) *Non-epileptic myoclonus.* Similar to that of the papio-papio, a photosensitive baboon with eyelid myoclonias (Menini *et al.*, 1994).

At this stage of our knowledge and understanding of these conditions, it is better to accept that we do not know the underlying mechanisms of these interesting phenomena. It would be premature and unhelpful to presume that these are attempts for self-induction. This is the most unlike explanation from all five possibilities listed above.

Why have the seizures of eyelid myoclonia have been mistaken as a manoeuvre for self-induction?

The first reports of photosensitive epilepsy were concerned with patients who had seizures when in bright sunlight or suddenly exposed to bright light or after exposure to bright sunlight for a period of time (Davidson & Watson, 1956; Robertson, 1954; Harding & Jeavons, 1994; Panayiotopoulos, 1972; 1995). In 1946 Gray Walter, using a high intensity lamp, found that intermittent photic stimulation could induce subjective and objective symptoms which correlated with specific EEG patterns and induced a 3 Hz generalized photoconvulsive response on a patient (Walter *et al.*, 1946). Gastaut in 1951 (quoted by Robertson, 1954) argued that intermittent photic stimulation was the responsible factor in inducing epileptic seizures and that any claims of observing seizure induction by continuous light should probably be discounted as due to interruptions of the light by flutter of the eyelids. Most modern epileptologists have unquestionably accepted that view and it is because of this they cannot accept eyelid myoclonia as a seizure elicited by uninterrupted light.

However, photosensitivity is not the only provocative factor in EMA. The most consistent and the most potent precipitating factors are associated with eye closure mechanisms to which very little attention has been paid (Panayiotopoulos, 1994; 1996a). Eye closure mechanisms and photosensitivity may be linked, the one enhancing the other, they often co-exist but they can also occur independently and the one may persist without the other. A similar situation may exist between eye closure which is mainly linked with photosensitivity and eyes-closed mechanisms which are mainly linked to fixation-off sensitivity (FOS). It is fascinating that two apparently opposite conditions (photosensitivity and FOS) can operate simultaneously as they do in some patients with EMA. EMA offers us a unique situation to study such mechanisms.

Conclusion

Eyelid myoclonia is an epileptic seizure (in patients with EMA). Eyelid myoclonia, may be a non-epileptic symptom in some patients with EMA but it should not be unquestionably equated with self-induction. Most likely, it is not.

We do not know the physiology of the epileptic phenomena and the alterations which may occur in the brain of patients with EMA under the continuous bombardment of electrical discharges when they close their eyes. Age of onset may be significant. This is the main challenge for further investigation.

Acknowledgements

We thank the Special Trustees of St. Thomas' Hospital for financial support for our studies on epilepsies.

References

Aicardi, J. (1994): *Epilepsy in children.* 2nd edition. *The international review of child neurology.* New York: Raven Press.

Antebi, D. & Bird, J. (1993): The facilitation and provocation of seizures. *Br. J. Psychiatry* **160**, 154–164.

Ames, F.R. (1971): Self-induction in photosensitive epilepsy. *Brain.* **94**, 781–798.

Ames, F.R. (1974): Cine film and EEG recordings during 'hand waving' in an epileptic photosensitive child. *Electroencephalogr. Clin. Neurophysiol.* **37**, 301–304.

Ames, F.R. & Saffer, D. (1983): The sunflower syndrome: a new look at 'self-induced' epilepsy. *J. Neurol. Sci.* **59**, 1–11.

Andermann, K. Oaks, G., Berman, S., Cooke, P.M., Dickson, J., Gastaut, H., Kennedy, A., Margerison, J., Pond, D.A., Tizard, J.P.M. & Walsh, E.G. ed. S.L. Sherwood (1962): Self-induced epilepsy. *Arch. Neurol.* **6**, 49–65.

Appleton, R.E., Panayiotopoulos, C.P., Acomb, B.A. & Beirne, M. (1993): Eyelid myoclonia with typical absences: an epilepsy syndrome. *J. Neurol. Neurosurg. Psychiatry* **56**, 1312–1316.

Asher, E.J. & Ort, R.S. (1951): Eye movements as a complex indication. *J. Gen. Psychol.* **45**, 209–217.

Bancaud, J. (1969): Les crises epileptiques d'origine occipitale (etude stereo-electroencephalographique). *Revue Otoneurophthalmol.* **41**, 299–315.

Binnie, C.D., Darby, C.E., de Korte, R.A. & Wilkins, A.J. (1980): Self-induction of epileptic seizures by eyeclosure: incidence and recognition. *J. Neurol. Neurosurg. Psychiatry* **43**, 386–389.

Binnie, C.D. & Jeavons, P.M. (1992): Photosensitive epilepsies. In: *Epileptic syndromes in infancy, childhood and adolescence,* edited by J. Roger, M. Bureau, Ch. Dravet, F.E. Dreifuss, A. Perret, P. Wolf. pp. 299–305. London: John Libbey.

Chao, D. (1962): Photogenic and self-induced epilepsy. *J. Pediatr.* **61**, 733–738.

Darby, C.E., de Korte, R.A., Binnie, C.D. & Wilkins, A.J. (1980): The self-induction of epileptic seizures by eye closure. *Epilepsia* **21**, 31–42.

Davidson, S. & Watson, C.W. (1956): Hereditary light-sensitive epilepsy. *Neurology* **6**, 235–261.

Duncan, J.S. & Panayiotopoulos, C.P. (1995): Typical absences with specific modes of precipitation (Reflex absences): Clinical aspects. In: *Typical absence seizures and related epileptic syndromes,* eds. J.S. Duncan & C.P. Panayiotopoulos, pp. 206–212. London: Churchill Livingstone.

Ferrie, C.D., De Marco, P., Grunewald, R.A., Giannakodimos, S. & Panayiotopoulos, C.P. (1994): Video-game induced seizures. *J. Neurol. Neurosurg. Psychiatry* **57,** 925–931.

Giannakodimos, S. & Panayiotopoulos, C.P. (1996): Eyelid myoclonia with absences in adults: a clinical and video-EEG study. *Epilepsia* (in press).

Green, J.B. (1966): Self-induced seizures: clinical and electroencephalographic studies. *Arch. Neurol.* **15,** 579–586.

Grünewald, R.A., Aliberti, V. & Panayiotopoulos, C.P. (1992): Exacerbation of typical absence seizures by progesterone. *Seizure* **1,** 137–138.

Harding, G.F.A. & Jeavons, P.M. (1994): *Photosensitive epilepsy.* 2nd edition. Clinics in Developmental Medicine **133,** London: Mac Keith Press.

Jeavons, P.M. (1977): Nosological problems of myoclonic epilepsies in childhood and adolescence. *Dev. Med. Child. Neurol.* **19,** 38.

Menini, C., Silva-Barrat, C. & Naquet, R. (1994): The epileptic and non epileptic generalized myoclonus in the Papio papio babbon. In: *Idiopathic generalized epilepsies: clinical, experimental and genetic aspects,* eds A. Malafosse, P. Genton, E. Hirsch, C. Marescaux, D. Broglin, R. Bernasconi R. pp. 331–348. London: John Libbey.

Munari, C., Bonis, A., Kochen, S., Pestre, M., *et al.* (1984): Eye movements and occipital seizures in man. *Acta Neurosurg.* **33,** (suppl) 47–52.

Panayiotopoulos, C.P. (1972): A study of photosensitive epilepsy with particular reference to occipital spikes induced by intermittent photic stimulation. Ph.D. Thesis. University of Aston, Birmingham.

Panayiotopoulos, C.P. (1979): Self-induced pattern sensitive epilepsy. *Arch. Neurol.* **36,** 48–50.

Panayiotopoulos, C.P. (1994): Fixation-off-sensitive epilepsies: clinical and EEG characteristics. In: *Epileptic seizures and syndromes,* ed., P. Wolf, pp. 55–65. London: John Libbey.

Panayiotopoulos, C.P. (1995): Epilepsies characterised by seizures with specific modes of precipitation (Reflex epilepsies). In: *Childhood epilepsy,* ed. S. Wallace. London: Chapman & Hall.

Panayiotopoulos, C.P. (1996a): Fixation-off sensitive, scotosensitive and other visual-related sensitive epilepsies. In: *Reflex epilepsies,* eds. S. Zifkin *et al.* New York: Raven Press (in press).

Panayiotopoulos, C.P. (1996b): Absence epilepsies: childhood, juvenile and myoclonic absence epilepsy, eyelid myoclonia with absences and other related epileptic syndromes with typical absence seizures. In: *Epilepsy: a comprehensive textbook,* eds., J.E. Engel & T.A. Pedley. (Volume 3, in press). New York: Raven Press.

Panayiotopoulos, C.P., Vasilopoulos, D. & Spengos, M. (1975): Self-induced epilepsy: clinical and electrophysiological study of a child. *Enkephalos.* **12,** 17–30.

Radovici, A., Misirliou, V. & Gluckman, M.L. (1932): Epilepsy reflexe provoquee par excitations optiques des rayons solaires. *Revue Neurologique* **1,** 1305–1307.

Rafal, R.D., Laxer, K.D. & Janowsky, J.S. (1986): Seizures triggered by blinking in a non-photosensitive epileptic. *J. Neurol. Neurosurg. Psychiatry* **49,** 445–447.

Robertson, E.G. (1954): Photogenic epilepsy: self-precipitated attacks. *Brain* **77,** 232–251.

Takeda, A., Bancaud, J. & Talairach, J. (1970): Concerning epileptic attacks of occipital origin. *Electroencephal. Clin. Neurophysiol.* **28,** 647.

Tassinari, C.A., Michelluci, R. & Rubboli, G. (1989): Self-induced seizures. In: *Reflex seizures and reflex epilepsies,* eds. A. Beaumanoir, H. Gastaut, R. Naquet, pp. 363–368. Geneva: Medecine & Hygiene.

Tassinari, C.A., Rubboli, G. & Michelluci, R. (1990): Reflex epilepsy. In: *Comprehensive epileptology,* eds. M. Dam & L. Gram, pp. 233–243. New York: Raven Press.

Walsh, F.B. (1957): *Clinical neuro-ophthalmology.* 2nd edition, pp. 186–245. Baltimore: The Williams & Wilkins Company.

Walter, W.G., Dovey, V.J. & Shipton, H. (1946): Analysis of the electrical response of the human cortex to photic stimulation. *Nature.* **158,** 540–541.

Wastell D.G., Wilkins, A.J. & Darby, C.E. (1982): Self-induction of epileptic seizures by eye-closure. Spectral analysis of concomitant EEG. *J. Neurol. Neurosurg. Psychiaty* **45,** 1151–1152.

Watanabe, K., Negoro, T., Matsumoto, A., Inokuma, M., Takaesu, E., Aso, K. & Yamamoto, N. (1985): Self-induced photogenic epilepsy in infants. *Arch. Neurol.* **42,** 406–407.

Williamson, P.D., Thadani, V.M., Darcey, T.M., Spencer, D.D., Spencer, S.S. & Mattson, R.H. (1992): Occipital lobe epilepsy: clinical characteristics, seizure spread patterns. and results of surgery. *Ann. Neurol.* **31,** 3–13.

Appendix

[1]Translation of the original paper reporting the first recorded case of EMA

Reflex epilepsy provoked by optic excitation by (means of) sunrays

M.M.A. Radovici, V.L. Misirliou and M. Gluckman

Bucarest, Hungary
Réunion Neurologique International, 31 Mai – 1er June 1932, pp. 1305–1308.

Reflex epilepsy is still considered as a pathological curiosity of, more or less, doubtful interpretation. A lesion of the motor cortex, in the first place, and distortion of the humoral balance are the two factors generally considered as sufficient to confirm the a pathogenesis of epilepsy. And yet, indisputable facts arise to demonstrate the determinant role that the afferent excitations sometimes may play through sensory, special sensory or vegetative pathways and the influence of the receptive cortical zones in triggering the convulsive attack. We think that we can expose an example of the kind in the following case.

Case history

A.A., 20 years old, admitted on the 20th of April 1931, presents motor disturbance in the form of involuntary movements of the head and eyes under the influence of sunlight. The initial manifestations date back approximately 10 years. At the age of 10–12, when he was still at primary school, his schoolfellows frequently frightened him by forcing him to gaze directly upwards. He claims that since then a tic has persisted consisting of head elevation mainly towards the sun. Rhythmic head movements with rotation in the direction of the sunlight were associated with fast eyelid blinking. This tic persisted also, though in much more attenuated form, during cloudy days. He has never manifested his tic after the sunset, in his room or in the artificial light of his apartment at night.

Since that date (10 years ago), the patient tells us that, from time to time and mainly during the summer when the sunlight is brighter, he has an exacerbation of his tic, resulting in paroxysms with falling and loss of consciousness. These crises occurred approximately two to three times per year. The tic of the head persisted between these paroxysmal attacks. Nothing was found to explain these manifestations on a heredofamilial base. There was no history of severe childhood illness, and no alcohol or tobacco abuse. Syphilis is denied. The mental state is fairly good. His physical structure is

---

1   *Translated from the original French paper by Dr. M. Koutroumanidis.*

moderate, rather weak and the thorax is carina-shaped. He has no active or passive motor deficit in the trunk or the extremities. Tendon and cutaneous reflexes are normal. The pupils are equal and reactive. Ocular motility is normal. No diplopia was claimed. No signs of parkinsonism are present. In both extreme lateral gaze positions, nystagmus is evident with fine horizontal and slightly rotatory oscillations. No nystagmus is observed in the extreme vertical positions. The general somatic sensation is preserved. Vision and hearing are normal. No abnormality was revealed from the neck, heart, lungs, gastrointestinal and genito-urinary systems. Examination of the vestibular system (Dr. Tetzu) by rotating and caloric induced vertigo, demonstrated a degree of labyrinthhyperexcitability.

We retained the patient in the clinic for two months for observation. Being perfectly normal from the psychic point of view, the patient gave us all the details of his affliction, without any tendency to exaggerate or to deceive. During cloudy days and generally when he was in the shadow, nothing could make one to suspect his 'mal' (disease), but from the time that he was outside under a sunny sky, he would start to present involuntary movements, of the head and eyes in the form of a salutatory tic with a varying frequency. This tic was consisting of a frequent and spasmodic blinking of the eyelids and of rhythmical movements, both rotating and elevating of the head towards the sun. The patient confessed that regarding his elevation tic, besides the attraction of the gaze by the sunlight, the influence of a psychic factor also exists. When he was with a person unknown to him or he was engaged in his own occupations, being absorbed by a (particular) aim to achieve, he forgot or perhaps subdued his tic. Alone and without occupation, walking round the streets, he would become the prey of his involuntary movements, thanks to (because of) which, by his characteristic gait with the head and eyes agitated by the sun, he became well known by his fellow citizens, in habitants of a small provincial town.

Willing to study in an analytical way and film the patient's solar tic, we placed him several times on a sunny terrace,at noon. The tic appeared straight away, becoming more and more accentuated both in terms of frequency and of amplitude of the movements of the head and the eyes. When the patient is forced to remain under these conditions, we were also able to observe the appearance of the paroxysms which are, typical of epileptic attacks. Artificial light – electric lamp, ultra-violet and infra-red light – does not trigger an attack. Because of the tic of the head and eyes towards the sun, which dominates the clinical picture, nobody had thought of the possibility of epilepsy. It is only during these provoked paroxysms that we realised that the spasmodic and rhythmic tic was in fact nothing but the start, self-restricted for the most of the time, of a generalized convulsive attack, which (though) from time to time was spontaneously evolving and could be experimentally provoked through violent optic excitation, due to sunlight.

We were able to capture characteristic successive moments from the beginning of the oculo-cephalic tic until the patient fell. At the time when the eyelid blinking and the head movements are maximal, a spiral, spasmodic torsion of the head and trunk is manifested, a saccadic groaning (follows) and the patient falls on the ground with generalized tonic-clonic convulsions. During the attack, the face and lips become cyanotic, there is foam in the mouth, the corneal reflexes and the overall somatic sensation is abolished. He loses consciousness and he is unable to recall the attack. He feels tired on recovery, has a headache and remains drowsy for the remaining of the day.

The patient tells us that he may abort (shrink away) these spontaneous paroxysms by placing the hand in front of the eyes and pressing down the eyelids with his fingers. During his admission, the patient had one spontaneous and two experimentally, (by exposing him to the sunlight), provoked convulsive attacks.

The conditions under which we have observed the patient and the study of his mental state, eliminate the hypothesis of simulation or of an hysterical manifestation. We have not been able to find in the literature other cases, similar to ours. However, it has been mentioned in the treatises on reflex epilepsy that, exceptionally, sensory excitations may trigger an epileptic attack. Recent data on experimental physiology substantiate a real base for the interpretation of these cases which seem rather strange at a first glance. Clementi from Florence has actually achieved to provoke convulsive attacks in dogs by means of optic, auditory and also olfactory excitations after strychnization of the respective sensory cortex. Considering the light in particular, its action on the overall nervous (system) excitability and conductibility has been recently evidenced by Achelis, Rosenberg and Sager. In our case – and this pertains in general in order to explain the reflex epilepsy – a local irritation of the sensory cortex could conduct focal strychnization and excite the cortical function in a way that afferent excitations could trigger convulsive attacks, starting always from the muscles of the corresponding area, which (muscles) in our case are the ocular of the eyelids, and (subsequently) becoming generalized.

References

A. Clementi (1929): *Arch. Fisiol.* **17,** (3). Strichninizazzione della sfera corticale visiva ed epilessia sperimentale da simoli luminosi.

A. Clementi. *Arch. f. Fisiol.,* t. (1931): XXX, no 1.

Van Ganegen. (1931): Crises epileptiform reflexes avec mouvements cephalo- et oculogyres par irritation des elements non sensoriels de l'oreille. *Ann. d'otolaryngologie* **69,** 9.

O. Foerster (1926): Die pathogenese der epileptischen Krampfanfalle. *Versamlung Deutscher Nervenarzt.*

Soli (1930): Crisi oculogire accompagnant de accesi epilettoidi un parkinsonian. *Giorn. Cl. Med.* **11.**

Achelis (1928): *Pflugers Arch.* **219.**

Faure Bealieu (1931): *Revue Neurologique* **11.**

Rosenberg & Sager (1931): *Pflugers Arch.* .**228.**

Chapter 13

Observations on families with eyelid myoclonia with absences

[1]A. Parker, [2]R.M. Gardiner, [3]C.P. Panayiotopoulos, [3]A. Agathonikou and [1]C.D. Ferrie

[1]*Department of Paediatric Neurology, Guy's Hospital, London;* [2]*The Rayne Institute, University College London Medical School;* [3]*Department of Clinical Neurophysiology and Epilepsies, St. Thomas' Hospital, London*

'From a family taint of the father, mother, relations or ancestor: the disease frequently lies dormant in the father, while it is derived from the grandfather to grandchild – Boerhaave (1668–1738) on the falling sickness ...'

The familial preponderance of epileptic disorders has been known since ancient times. It was because of this and social prejudice that even in the latter half of the twentieth century people with epileptic disorders were forcibly sterilized in Germany (Conrad, 1939) or forbidden from marriage unless sterilized in Sweden (Alstrom, 1951).

Early studies quote widely differing incidence in affected relatives. The discrepancy was due to different diagnostic criteria and later to the inclusion/exclusion of EEG findings.

It is only recently that precise definitions and classifications, a prerequisite for genetic studies, have been used. The International League Against Epilepsy (ILAE) has published a proposal for the classification of epilepsies and epileptic syndromes (Commission on Classification and Terminology, 1989) which is based on observations of clinicians. The identification of epileptic syndromes (clusters of clinical and EEG features which are associated in a non-fortuitous manner, and which may represent distinct disease aetiologies) is an important medical advance for the diagnosis, management and genetic investigation of epilepsies (Grunewald & Panayiotopoulos, 1996). Some parts of the ILEA classification remain contentious, some syndromes are ill- or broadly defined and require further clarification. There are patients whose clinical and EEG features do not appear to fit neatly into any recognized category or erroneously appear to 'evolve' from one syndrome to another. Some may represent new or overlap syndromes, others may be unusual forms of known syndromes or cases where clinical history is misleading (Grunewald & Panayiotopoulos, 1996).

The investigation of epilepsies cannot take advantage of the advances in molecular genetics without a firm definition of possible phenotypes in particular epileptic syndromes. When this has been possible (benign familial neonatal convulsions, Baltic and Mediterranean progressive myoclonic epilepsy) significant progress has been made in identifying gene locus.

Idiopathic generalized epilepsies (IGE), which are probably genetically determined, comprise several different and possibly unrelated conditions despite some superficial resemblance (Panayiotopoulos, 1995; Malafosse *et al.*, 1994a) and the hypothesis of a biological continuum (Berkovic *et al.*, 1987; 1994; Andermann; 1995).

Eyelid myoclonia with absences (EMA), may be suitable for future genetic molecular studies as it appears to be a distinct form of idiopathic generalized epilepsies with the triad of eyelid myoclonia with absences, eye closure provocation of seizures or EEG paroxysms, and photosensitivity constituting the syndrome of EMA. This is a preliminary study of families with EMA.

Materials and methods

In the last 5 years, we have seen 15 adults and three children with strict clinical-EEG criteria of eyelid myoclonia with absences. Sixteen were female. Our methods for studying these patients are described in Chapters 6 & 8. All but four patients had a positive family history of epileptic seizures. In four families positive histories for a similar condition (EMA) affecting other family members were obtained.

Clinical examination and video EEG recordings were requested from relatives who were possibly affected but in only three this was possible. In all others the information is based on description by other members of the families, and previous medical reports and EEGs.

Clinical examination and EEG recording were not requested in family members without a history of abnormality of eyelid movement or seizures.

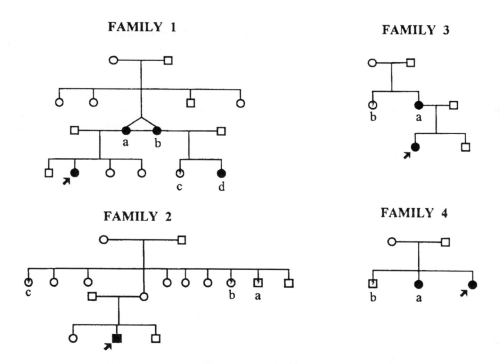

Fig. 1. Families with proband with eyelid myoclonia and absences. Proband (arrow), EMA (filled square or circle), eyelid closure abnormality/other absence syndrome (question mark).

Results

The four probands had 11 first or second degree relatives with seizures or clinically apparent transient eyelid movements (Fig. 1).

Family 1

The proband born in 1985 is described in detail as case 1 in Chapter 6. Briefly, she was normal until aged 4 when she developed eyelid myoclonia with absences exacerbated by sunlight. Video EEG confirmed the diagnosis of EMA.

The mother (a) and aunt (b) of the proband are identical twins born in 1959. They both had normal development until aged nine when eyelid myoclonia with absences started. Like the proband these were exacerbated by sunlight and television. They both developed generalized tonic-clonic seizures as teenagers. The mother (a) had video-EEG confirmation of EMA and remains photosensitive. The aunt (c) refused video-EEG but previous EEG showed generalized polyspike and spike/slow wave discharges on eye closure, particularly during photic stimulation. Some of the discharges were associated with limb myoclonic jerks.

The proband's cousin (c), born in 1984, was normal until the age of 8 years when she developed frequent typical absences with severe impairment of consciousness and without reported ictal eyelid manifestations. She was not photosensitive. An EEG was reported as showing two seizures of 3 Hz generalized discharges of spike and wave during hyperventilation. They lasted for 20 s 'during which the child was unresponsive, opened her eyes and spontaneously stopped hyperventilation'. Absences were controlled with ethosuximide.

Cousin (d) born in 1981 developed absences, eyelid fluttering, generalized tonic-clonic seizures and photosensitivity at age 7 years. Symptoms improved with sodium valproate, generalized tonic-clonic seizures and the seizures stopped, but she continues having absences and eyelid fluttering. Sleep deprivation EEG showed generalized spike/polyspike and wave discharges on eye closure and photoconvulsive responses. There was a dramatic increase of the discharges on awakening. We classified cousin (d) as EMA despite lack of video-EEG.

Family 2

The proband born in 1987 was normal until aged 7 years when he developed daytime enuresis. His mother noted that he looked 'absent' during these episodes. Video-EEG showed eyelid myoclonia with absences and photosensitivity. His uncle (a) born in 1956 was normal until developing absences with 'eyelid fluttering' and frequent generalized tonic-clonic seizures at age 9 years. He was not controlled on phenobarbitone, phenytoin and ethosuximide. generalized tonic-clonic seizures and absences continue in adulthood. His school progress was poor and he later served multiple prison terms. Previous EEG reports and recordings were obtained from the age of 14 years. These showed brief and long generalized discharges of 2.5–4 Hz spike and polyspikes. Eyelid fluttering was noted in some of them. In only the initial EEG was some evidence of photosensitivity reported.

Aunt (b) born in 1960 had a history of photosensitivity , absences, eyelid 'fluttering' and generalized tonic-clonic seizures.

Aunt (c) born in 1969 also had a history of absences and photosensitivity from the age of eight.

No more details and no medical records could be obtained for aunt (b) and (c).

Family 3

The proband born in 1974 presented at the age of 4 years with eyelid myoclonia with absences associated with retropulsion of the head and photosensitivity. She developed coeliac disease as a child. The absences continued throughout childhood despite treatment with sodium valproate. She had spontaneous generalized tonic-clonic seizures and myoclonic jerks, which were also photically evoked. They were more frequent on awakening and during menstruation. On referral to us at 19 years of age, during the interview she had numerous episodes of eyelid myoclonia particularly when looking at bright sunlight and on eye closure. The diagnosis of EMA was confirmed with video EEG which showed brief generalized discharges mainly on eye closure. These were associated with small range eyelid jerking. She was highly photosensitive.

Her mother (a) born in 1948, gave a history of eyelid fluttering and frequent TV-induced generalized tonic-clonic seizures from the age of 11 years. Initial treatment with phenobarbitone was unsuccessful, phenytoin was better, but, did not completely abolish the absences and the eyelid fluttering which continues. Video EEG was compatible with EMA. Only occipital spikes were elicited by IPS.

The aunt (b) declined EEG, but had a history of marked eyelid fluttering, absences and photosensitivity with onset at the same age as her sister.

Family 4

The proband born in 1953 (case 2 in Giannakodimos & Panayiotopoulos, 1996) was normal until she developed eyelid myoclonia with absences at age 10 years, with three TV-induced generalized tonic-clonic seizures.

Her sister (a) born in 1949 (case 3 in Giannakodimos & Panayiotopoulos, 1996) presented after EMA was diagnosed in the proband. She started having eyelid myoclonia with absences at age 7 years and generalized tonic-clonic seizures (mainly TV-induced and catamenial) aged 11 years. She remained well controlled until the recurrence of nocturnal generalized tonic-clonic seizures aged 35 years. She continues to have eyelid myoclonia. In both sisters EMA was confirmed on video EEG.

Their brother (b) born in 1957 developed absences, generalized tonic-clonic seizures and occasional myoclonic jerks aged 10 years. He was not photosensitive. He declined video EEG. An EEG at age 15 years was reported as showing 'frequent generalized theta activity at 4–7 Hz more markedly post-centrally, intermittently associated with sharp waves. This was reduced by visual stimuli. Generalized, brief, atypical spike and wave activity occurred during hyperventilation'.

The mother developed symptomatic complex seizures due to cerebrovascular disease, and her video-EEG showed only diffuse slow activity.

The affected individuals in these four families had high concordance of clinical type of idopathic generalized epilepsy. Sixty per cent had EMA, 80 per cent were photosensitive and possibly all had absences. Only three patients did not show evidence of photosensitivity.

Discussion

This preliminary study gives an insight into the familial preponderance of EMA. It is not possible to draw firm conclusions as unaffected relatives were not examined and video EEG recordings were not obtained from all the affected relatives. The questions of incidence of epileptiform abnormalities and their penetrance remained unanswered.

In family 1, the proband, her mother and the maternal homozygous twin sister have identical symptoms characteristic of EMA: eyelid myoclonia with absences, EEG discharges precipitated by eye closure and photosensitivity. The same is probably true for her cousin (d), but cousin (c) has prolonged typical absences without eyelid myoclonia, eye closure EEG paroxysms and photosensitivity. Cousin (c), based on the available information, could be classified as childhood or juvenile absence epilepsy according to ILAE criteria.

In family 2, the proband has clinical and EEG evidence of EMA. It is also possible that the two maternal aunts had EMA but this is based only on clinical information of 'absences with eyelid fluttering and photosensitivity' which is inadequate and may be biased. The maternal uncle (a) is difficult to classify despite reports of absences with eyelid fluttering. He may not have photosensitivity despite the initial EEG report.

In family 3, the proband and mother had EMA. There were variations in clinical type; the daughter was brought to medical attention because of eyelid myoclonia and absences, while the mother's initial problem were TV-induced generalized tonic-clonic seizures. However, the proband's detailed medical notes did not make reference to the eyelid myoclonia, which was both frequent and violent during her first interview with us at age 19 years. Maternal aunt (b) may also have EMA, and her disease is recognised by her sister as identical.

In family 4, the proband and her sister have been thoroughly investigated and the diagnosis of EMA is firmly established. Their brother (b) was not photosensitive and there was no history of eyelid myoclonia, a symptom of which his sisters are well aware. Based on the available information one could possibly force a diagnosis of juvenile absence epilepsy or juvenile myoclonic epilepsy. However, an EEG at age 15 indicates that the abnormalities were mainly on eyes-closed which may be an indication of fixation-off sensitivity from which his sisters also suffered.

Thus, in this limited study, allowing for decisions regarding affected members for whom descriptions and previous medical/EEG reports were the only available source of information, the following conclusions can be reached:

(a) There are families with a strong prevalence of all manifestations of EMA, as defined by us, amongst affected members. There were nine definite cases of EMA amongst the 15 affected members.

(b) All but three patients, had clinical and/or EEG photosensitivity.

(c) EEG eye closure precipitation of EEG paroxysms occurred in all but three patients, from those in whom EEGs were available.

(d) There is a strong female preponderance (12 out of 15 affected members). In two families (1 and 3) only female members were affected. Paternal inheritance was not evident in the three families with more than one generation affected.

(e) There were two definite cases in which a syndrome other than EMA was established (case c of family 1 and case b of family 4).

(f) All patients appear to have absences.

Bianchi *et al.* (1995), in their study group of families with more than one member affected by a form of idiopathic generalized epilepsies, reported concordance in clinical syndromes of relatives of probands with childhood absence epilepsy in which no incidence of EMA was found. Conversely, they also reported concordance of syndrome in families of probands with EMA and suggested that their data indicate a different clinical and genetic basis for childhood absence epilepsy and other epilepsies with absences and photosensitivity, in particular juvenile myoclonic epilepsy and EMA.

Bianchi *et al.* (1995) also reported three families of probands with 'absences, myoclonia, generalized tonic-clonic seizures and photosensitivity'. In the first family, two sisters were affected. The father and the paternal grandfather had 'epilepsy with generalized tonic-clonic seizures'. The proband of the second family was a girl, her father and a cousin also had 'epilepsy with generalized tonic-clonic seizures'. The proband of the third family was a boy, the maternal father had 'epilepsy with generalized tonic-clonic seizures'.

Four other probands had 'childhood absence epilepsy with eyelid myoclonia'. The proband of the first family was a girl, the mother was diagnosed as having juvenile myoclonic epilepsy and a cousin as having 'absences, myoclonia, generalized tonic-clonic seizures and photosensitivity'. The proband of the second family, his twin brother and their sister had 'childhood absence epilepsy with eyelid myoclonia'. The mother had 'epilepsy with generalized tonic-clonic seizures'. The proband of the third family was a girl, her mother had 'epilepsy with generalized tonic-clonic seizures' and her brother had febrile convulsions. The proband of the fourth family was a girl, her maternal aunt, uncle and grandmother had 'epilepsy with generalized tonic-clonic seizures'.

There was no case of 'childhood absence epilepsy with eyelid myoclonia' or 'absences, myoclonia, generalized tonic-clonic seizures and photosensitivity' in the 24 families of probands with childhood absence epilepsy and three with juvenile absence epilepsy.

Thus, EMA in these families, appears as a homogeneous syndrome which may be genetically independent from some idiopathic generalized epilepsies. Links with other idiopathic generalized epilepsies cannot be excluded, particularly those manifesting with absences and/or photosensitivity and/or epileptic disorders with eye closure induced abnormalities

Patients with juvenile myoclonic epilepsy by definition have myoclonic jerks; 80 per cent of them also suffer from generalized tonic-clonic seizures, one third have absences, photosensitivity occurs in 33 per cent and eye closure induced EEG discharges have been reported (Grunewald & Panayiotopoulos, 1993; Panayiotopoulos, 1994; Panayiotopoulos et al., 1994). Despite common clinical manifestations between juvenile myoclonic epilepsy and EMA we have not seen the characteristic eyelid myoclonic seizures of EMA in over 150 strictly defined patients with juvenile myoclonic epilepsy (Panayiotopoulos, 1994; 1996b). Juvenile myoclonic epilepsy is the first idiopathic generalized epilepsies for which evidence of linkage was reported, with serological markers on chromosome 6p (HLA loci and properdin factor Bf locus EJM1). This linkage has not been confirmed by other investigators, which may be explained by locus heterogeneity (Anderson & Rich, 1994; Anderson et al., 1994a; Delgado-Escueta et al., 1990; 1994; Greenberg et al., 1988; Whitehouse et al., 1993; Gardiner, 1995; Anderman, E., 1995). An interesting group of families with autosomally inherited juvenile myoclonic epilepsy has been described in Saudi Arabia where consanguinity is high, these patients may be valuable when investigated with molecular genetic techniques (Panayiotopoulos & Obeid, 1989).

In a comparative genetic study between juvenile myoclonic epilepsy and generalized tonic clonic seizures on awakening (Igeneralized tonic-clonic seizuresA), Greenberg et al. (1995) showed a significant difference in the incidence of two HLA groups, DR13 and DQb1, between a group of patients with juvenile myoclonic epilepsy and a similar sized group with IGTCSA. This implies different inheritance between these two diseases. Genetic studies in patients with typical absences have failed so far to show linkage with a particular chromosome (Gardiner, 1995; Andermann, E., 1995; Sanders et al., 1993) which may be attributed to the lack of precise phenotypic definitions (Panayiotopoulos, 1995; Panayiotopoulos, 1996b). In animals with absences there is confirmed linkage with many chromosomes (Noebels, 1994; 1995).

Regarding photosensitivity, it should be emphasized that photosensitivity is not one disease and this clinical and/or EEG trait can be found in many unrelated epileptic conditions, most of which have a strong genetic element (Waltz, 1994; Panayiotopoulos, 1996a; also Daly & Bickford, 1951; Davidson & Watson, 1957; Delgado-Escueta et al., 1987; Doose & Waltz, 1993).

Photosensitivity is common (90 per cent) in the Baltic/Mediterranean progressive myoclonic epilepsy for which genetic linkage with chromosome 21p 22.3 (locus EPM1) has been documented (Malafosse et al., 1994b; Anderson et al, 1994). Photosensitivity is also a feature of the type 3 juvenile form of Gaucher's disease and the gene for the deficient enzyme glucocerebrosidase has been mapped to q21q31 of chromosome 1 (Barnveld et al., 1983).

Eye closure EEG abnormalities without photosenitivity are common in patients with chromosome 4p syndrome (Sgro et al., 1995).

The significance of an accurate phenotypic definition for genetic analysis has been recently demonstrated in a newly described syndrome of autosomal dominant nocturnal frontal lobe epilepsy, characterized by brief violent hyperkinetic or tonic seizures after falling asleep or in the early morning, with onset in childhood. An autosomal dominant inheritance has been identified in five families and showed linkage with chromosome 20q13.2 in one but not the other four families (Berkovic *et al.*, 1995).

Future direction

In these families EMA appears to be a discrete syndrome of idiopathic generalized epilepsies with striking clinical and EEG features, strong familial preponderance and high concordance. Our preliminary study indicates that there may be families with EMA suitable for molecular genetic analysis. The phenotypic expressions of EMA with symptoms common with other idiopathic generalized epilepsies (localized and limb myoclonia; absences; photosensitivity; eye closure precipitation of seizures and EEG paroxysms; generalized tonic-clonic seizures often catamenial, on awakening or precipitated by sleep deprivation and fatigue) may help in better defining other idiopathic generalized epilepsies (by applying exclusion criteria) and make them more suitable for genetic analysis.

References

Alstrom, CH. (1951): *A study of epilepsy and its clinical, social and genetic aspects.* Stockholm: Ejnar Munksgaard .

Andermann, E. (1995): The genetics of typical absences-future directions-consensus statement. In: *Typical absences and related epileptic syndromes,* edited by J.S. Duncan & C.P. Panayiotopoulos. pp. 338–343. London: Churchill Livingstone.

Andermann, F. (1995): Typical absences are all part of the same disease. In: *Typical absences and related epileptic syndromes,* eds. J.S. Duncan and C.P. Panayiotopoulos. pp. 300–304. London: Churchill Livingstone.

Anderson, V.E. & Rich, S.S. (1994): Mapping epilepsy genes: a bridge between clinical and genetic studies. In: *Epileptic seizures and syndromes,* eds. P. Wolf. pp. 183–192. London: John Libbey.

Anderson, V.E., Leppert, M., Lindhoot, D., Malafosse, A. & Steinlein, O. (1994): Gene mapping for benign familial neonatal convulsions and related syndromes. In: *Idiopathic generalized epilepsies: clinical, experimental and genetic aspects,* edited by A. Malafosse, P. Genton, E. Hirsch, C. Marescaux, D. Broglin, R. Bernasconi. pp. 65–71. London: John Libbey.

Barneveld, R.A., Kiejzer, W., Tegelaers, F., Ginns, E., Gewrts Van Knessel, A., Brady, R.O. (1983): Assignment of the gene for human β-glucocerebroside to the region of q21q31 of chromosome 1 using monoclonal antibodies. *Hum. Gen.* **64,** 227–231.

Berkovic, S. (1994). Epilepsies in twins. In: *Epileptic seizures and syndromes,* edited by P. Wolf. pp.157–164. London: John Libbey.

Berkovic, S.F., Andermann, F., Andermann, E. & Gloor, P. (1987): Concepts of absence epilepsies: discrete syndromes or biological continuum? *Neurology* **37,** 993–1000.

Berkovic, S.F, Reutens, D.C., Andermann, E. & Andermann, F. (1994): The epilepsies: specific syndromes or a neurobiological continuum? In: *Epileptic seizures and syndromes,* eds. P. Wolf. pp. 25–37. London: John Libbey.

Berkovic, S.F., Phillips, H.A., Scheffer, I.E., Lopes-Cendes, I., Bhatia, K.P. & Fish, D.R. (1995): Genetic heterogeneity in autosomal dominant nocturnal frontal lobe epilepsy. *Epilepsia* **36** (suppl 4), 147.

Bianchi, A. and the Italian League Against Epilepsy Collaborative Group (1995): Study of concordance of symptoms in families with absence epilepsies. In: *Typical absences and related epileptic syndromes,* eds J.S.Duncan and C.P. Panayiotopoulos, pp. 328–337. London: Churchill Livingstone.

Commission on Classification and Terminology of the International League Against Epilepsy (1989): Proposal for classification of epilepsies and epileptic syndromes. *Epilepsia* **30,** 389–399.

Conrad, K. (1940): *Die erbliche fallsucht.* vol. 3. Leipzig: Ed Gutt.

Daly, D. & Bickford, R.G. (1951): Electroencephalographic studies of identical twins with photosensitivity. *EEG. Clin.Neurophysiol.* **3,** 378.

Davidson, D. & Watson, C.W. (1957): Hereditary light sensitive epilepsy. *Neurology* **6,** 235–261.

Delgado-Escueta, A.V., Abad Herrera, P., Treiman, L., Maldonado, I.I., Greenberg, D.A., Schwartz, B.E. (1987): Clinical and EEG phenotypes of early childhood photic and self-induced epilepsy: five generations in one pedigree. *Epilepsia* **28,** 584–585.

Delgado-Escueta, A.V., Greenberg, D.A., Weissbecker, K.A., Lin, A., Treiman, L., Sparkes, R., Park, M.S., Barbetti, A., Terasaki, P.I. (1990): Gene mapping in the idiopathic generalized epilepsies: juvenile myoclonic epilepsy, childhood absence epilepsy, epilepsy with grand mal seizures and early childhood myoclonic epilepsy. *Epilepsia* (suppl). **31,** S19–S29.

Doose, H., Waltz, S. (1993): Photosensitivity-genetics and clinical significance. *Neuropediatrics* **24,** 249–255.

Gardiner, M. (1995): Genetics of human typical absence syndromes. In: *Typical absences and related epileptic syndromes,* eds. J.S. Duncan and C.P. Panayiotopoulos. pp. 320–327. London: Churchill Livingstone.

Giannakodimos, S., Panayiotopoulos, C.P. (1996): Eyelid myoclonia with absences in adults: a clinical video-EEG study. *Epilepsia* **37,** 36–45.

Greenberg, D.A., Delgado-Escueta, A.V., Widelitz, H. *et al.*. (1988): Juvenile myoclonic epilepsy may be linked to the Bf and HLA loci on human chromosome 6. *Am. J. Med. Genet.* **31,** 185–192.

Greenberg, D.A., Durner, M., Shinnar, S. & Rosenbaum, D. (1995): HLADR and DQ alleles show an association with JME compared to non-JME forms of idiopathic generalized epilepsies. *Epilepsia* **36,** (suppl 4) 147.

Grunewald, R.A. & Panayiotopoulos, C.P. (1993): Juvenile myoclonic epilepsy: a review. *Arch. Neurol.* **50,** 594–598.

Grunewald, R.A. & Panayiotopoulos, C.P. (1996): The diagnosis of epilepsies. *J.R. Coll. Physicians Lond.* **30,** 122–127.

Malafosse, A., Genton, P., Hirsch, E., Marescaux, C., Broglin, D. & Bernasconi R. (1994a). Introduction. In: *Idiopathic generalized epilepsies: clinical, experimental and genetic aspects,* eds. A. Malafosse, P. Genton, E. Hirsch, C. Marescaux, D. Broglin & R. Bernasconi. pp. xvii. London: John Libbey.

Malafosse, A., Mandel, J.-L., Greenberg, D. & Baldy-Moulinier, M. (1994b): Molecular and statistical methods for mapping human epilepsy genes. In: *Idiopathic generalized epilepsies: clinical, experimental and genetic aspects,* eds. A. Malafosse, P. Genton, E. Hirsch, C. Marescaux, D. Broglin & R. Bernasconi. pp. 27–36. London: John Libbey.

Noebels, J.L. (1994): Genetic and phenotypic heterogeneity of inherited spike-and-wave epilepsies. In: *Idiopathic generalized epilepsies: clinical, experimental and genetic aspects,* edited by A. Malafosse, P. Genton, E. Hirsch, C. Marescaux, D. Broglin, R. & Bernasconi R. pp. 215–225. London: John Libbey.

Noebels, J.L. (1995): Genetic mechanisms of spike wave epilepsies in mouse mutants. In: *Typical absences and related epileptic syndromes,* eds. J.S. Duncan & C.P. Panayiotopoulos. pp. 29–38. London: Churchill Livingstone.

Panayiotopoulos, C.P. (1994): Juvenile myoclonic epilepsy: an underdiagnosed syndrome. In: *Epileptic seizures and syndromes,* ed. P. Wolf, pp. 221–230. London: John Libbey.

Panayiotopoulos C.P. (1995): Typical absences are syndrome-related. In: *Typical absences and related epileptic syndromes,* eds. J.S. Duncan & C.P. Panayiotopoulos, pp. 304–314. London: Churchill Livingstone,.

Panayiotopoulos, C.P. (1996a): Epilepsies characterised by seizures with specific modes of precipitation (Reflex epilepsies). In: *Childhood Epilepsy,* ed. S. Wallace, pp. 355–375. London: Chapman & Hall.

Panayiotopoulos C.P. (1996b): Absence epilepsies: childhood, juvenile and myoclonic absence epilepsy, eyelid myoclonia with absences and other related epileptic syndromes with typical absence seizures. In: *Epilepsy,* eds. J. Engel & T.A. Pedley. New York: Raven Press. (in press).

Panayiotopoulos, C.P. & Obeid, T. (1989): Juvenile myoclonic epilepsy: an autosomal disease. *Ann. Neurol.* **25,** 440–443.

Panayiotopoulos, C.P. Obeid, T. & Tahan, A. (1994): Juvenile myoclonic epilepsy: a 5 year prospective study. *Epilepsia* **35,** 285–296.

Sanders, T., Hildmann, T., Janz, M.D., Wienker,T.F., Neitzel, H., Bianchi, A., Bauer, G., Sailer, U., Berek, K., Schmitz, B. & Beck-Managetta, G. (1993): The phenotypic spectrum related to the human susceptibility gene 'EJM1'. *Ann. Neurol.* **38,** 210–217.

Sgro, V., Riva, E., Canevini, M.P., Colamaria, V., Rottoli, A., Minotti, O., Canger, R., Dalla Bernadina, B. (1995): 4p-syndrome: a chromosomal disorder associated with a particular EEG pattern. *Epilepsia* **36,**. 1206–1214.

Waltz, S. (1994): Photosensitivity and epilepsy: a genetic approach. In: *Idiopathic generalized epilepsies: clinical, experimental and genetic aspects,* edited by A. Malafosse, P. Genton, E. Hirsch, C. Marescaux, D. Broglin, R. Bernasconi, pp. 317–328. London: John Libbey.

Whitehouse, W.P., Rees, M., Curtis, D., Sundqvist, A., Parker, K., Chung, E., Baralle, D., Gardiner, R.M. (1993): Linkage analysis of idiopathic generalized epilepsies and marker loci on chromosome 6p in families of patients with juvenile myoclonic epilepsy: no evidence for an epilepsy locus in the HLA region. *Am. J. Hum. Genet* **53**, 652–662.

Eyelid Myoclonia with Absences, edited by J.S. Duncan and C.P. Panayiotopoulos
© 1996 John Libbey & Company Ltd, pp. 117–120.

Chapter 14

Treatment of eyelid myoclonia with absences

Alan Richens

Department of Pharmacology & Therapeutics, University of Wales College of Medicine, Heath Park, Cardiff, CF4 4XN, UK

Although Jeavons defined eyelid myoclonia with absences (EMA) as a specific entity in 1977 (Jeavons, 1977), it has not commonly been separated from other types of absence seizures and has not therefore been the subject of formal therapeutic trials, either controlled or uncontrolled. Investigators with the most clinical experience of this syndrome describe it as more difficult to control than typical absences or other types of idiopathic generalized epilepsy (De Marco 1989; Appleton *et al.* 1993) and it may persist into adult life. Although accompanying generalized tonic-clonic seizures may respond well to drug therapy, the eyelid myoclonia and associated absences may be refractory.

Appleton *et al.* (1993) described five children with this condition. Carbamazepine and phenytoin treatment resulted in either no improvement or a deterioration in seizure control. Valproate or ethosuximide produced a partial response in four, but the best results were obtained with a combination of these two drugs. In the four children in whom this combination was tried, seizures were abolished or dramatically reduced. Appleton (1995) concluded that sodium valproate in combination with either ethosuximide (Appleton *et al.* 1993) or occasionally clobazam (De Marco, 1989) appeared to be more effective in treating this condition than if a single drug is used. One patient was reported to have responded to a combination of lamotrigine and sodium valproate (Appleton, 1995).

Other types of absence seizures

In the absence of therapeutic trials in EMA it might be helpful to review briefly the preferred treatment of other epileptic syndromes involving absence seizures. This topic recently was reviewed by three investigators at an earlier symposium (Richens, 1995; Gram, 1995; Chadwick, 1995).

Many studies of ethosuximide and valproate, mostly uncontrolled, showed that both drugs were effective in reducing absence seizure frequency, sometimes achieving complete seizure control. Unfortunately, many of the studies of ethosuximide were undertaken before the international classifications of seizures and epilepsies were published and it is therefore difficult to know what types of absence seizures were included. Four comparative studies involving a total of 93 patients showed similar response rates to the two drugs (Richens, 1995). It was concluded that the choice

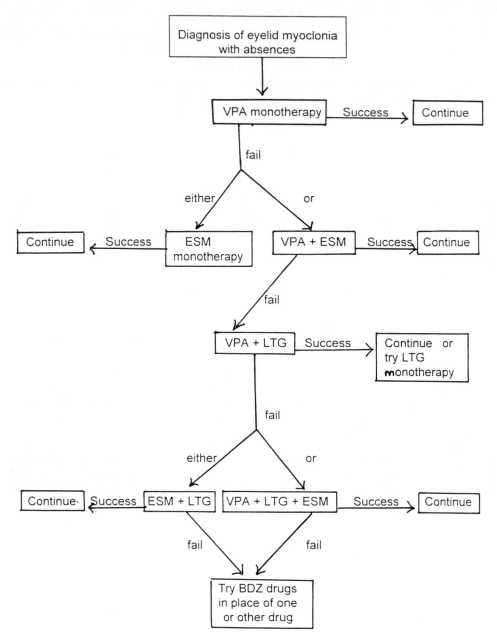

Fig 1. An algorithm suggesting a suitable approach to the treatment of eyelid myoclonia with absences. VPA = valproate, ESM = ethosuximide, LTG = lamotrigine, BDZ = benzodiazepine drugs.

of drug should depend upon whether or not other seizure types coexisted, sodium valproate having a broad spectrum of efficacy compared with ethosuximide's more specific action. It was noted that a combination of the two drugs would sometimes be effective where each drug alone had been unsatisfactory (Rowan *et al.* 1983).

Acetazolamide, benzodiazepine drugs and lamotrigine were considered to be second line treatments, to be used when sodium valproate or ethosuximide alone or in combination had failed (Gram, 1995). As lamotrigine had been introduced into European practice for only a relatively short period of time, and had not been widely studied in idiopathic generalized epilepsies, the position of this drug was uncertain. An update is therefore given below.

Gabapentin and felbamate were considered to have no place in the treatment of absence seizures on the evidence available (Chadwick, 1995).

Lamotrigine

An early analysis of the results of 27 non-comparative trials of lamotrigine in 572 patients showed that just over half of the 24 patients with typical absences and just under half of those 11 with atypical absences had a 50 per cent or greater reduction in seizure frequency with lamotrigine (Richens & Yuen, 1991). One third of the 11 patients with myoclonic seizures achieved the same result. In a preliminary communication Sander *et al.* (1991) noted that refractory absence seizures appeared to respond more favourably to lamotrigine than other seizure types, one of 19 patients becoming seizure-free. Myoclonic seizures improved in two of seven patients.

Gibbs *et al.* (1992) also published a preliminary communication in which all of four patients with intractable atypical absences showed a 50 per cent or greater reduction in seizure frequency with lamotrigine therapy, and myoclonic seizures in two of seven patients were also decreased in frequency.

Using a spike-and-wave monitor to record seizure frequency, Besag (1992; 1994) showed that lamotrigine appears to be remarkably effective in suppressing spike-and-wave events in children with intractable seizures.

Schlumberger *et al.* (1994) also describe their clinical experience with lamotrigine in 120 children, nine of whom had absences and another nine had myoclonic absences. At the end of 3 months treatment seven of the children with absences and four of those with myoclonic absences had shown a 50 per cent or greater reduction in seizure frequency. These results were considered to be most encouraging in that all the patients had previously received a combination of valproate and ethosuximide, but their seizures had proved resistant. Particularly notable was the response of myoclonic absences, a difficult syndrome to control with drug therapy. Similar results have been shown by Manonmani & Wallace (1994), who found that six children with this condition responded well (a 75 per cent or greater reduction in seizure frequency) to a combination of lamotrigine and ethosuximide or valproate, when they had failed to respond to the latter two drugs. A combination of lamotrigine and valproate has also been found to be particularly rewarding in patients with intractable typical and atypical absences (Panayiotopoulos *et al.* 1993; Ferrie & Panayiotopoulos, 1994) and in a single patient with EMA (Appleton, 1995).

The clinical experience of Buchanan (1995) is similar in that four of his eight patients with refractory absences became seizure-free on lamotrogine as add-on therapy. He observed also that the seizures of juvenile myoclonic epilepsy responded well in patients who were unable to tolerate sodium valproate, in agreement with an earlier report by Timmings & Richens (1992).

Conclusion

In the absence of controlled therapeutic trials it is not possible to draw scientifically valid conclusions on the most effective approach to the drug treatment of EMA. Based on the anecdotal evidence available in this condition, together with more objective results from trials in related absence syndromes, a scheme is suggested in Fig 1. It is possible, however, that lamotrigine will move up in priority when the results of further trials are available, perhaps supplanting ethosuximide. The possible role of other new drugs, for example topiramate, will need to be assessed.

References

Appleton, R.E. (1995): Eyelid myoclonia with absences. In *Typical absences and related epileptic syndromes*, eds J.S. Duncan & C.P. Panayiotopoulos, pp. 213–220. London: Churchill Livingstone.

Appleton, R.E., Panayiotopoulos, C.P., Acomb, B.A. & Beirne, M. (1993): Eyelid myoclonia with typical absences: an epilepsy syndrome. *J. Neurol. Neurosurg. Psychiatry* **56**, 1312–316.

Besag, F. (1992). Lamotrigine: paediatric experience. In *Clinical update on lamotrigine: a new antiepileptic agent*, ed A. Richens, pp. 53–60. Tunbridge Wells: Wells Medical.

Besag, F.M.C. (1994). Lamotrigine in the management of subtle seizures. *Rev. Contemp. Pharmacother.* **5**, 123–131.

Buchanan, N. (1995). Lamotrigine: clinical experience in 93 patients with epilepsy. *Acta Neurol. Scand.* **92**, 28–32.

Chadwick, D. (1995). Gabapentin and felbamate. In *Typical absences and related epileptic syndromes*, eds J.S. Duncan & C.P. Panayiotopoulos, pp. 213–220. London: Churchill Livingstone.

De Marco, P. (1989): Eyelid myoclonia with absences (EMA) in two monovular twins. *Clin. Electroencephalogr.* **20**, 193–195.

Ferrie, C.D. & Panayiotopoulos, C.P. (1994): Therapeutic interaction of lamotrigine and sodium valproate in intractable myoclonic epilepsy. *Seizure* **3**, 157–159.

Gibbs, J., Appleton, R.E., Rosenbloom, L. & Yuen, W.C. (1992): Lamotrigine for intractable childhood epilepsy: a preliminary communication. *Dev. Med. Child Neurol.* **34**, 369–371.

Gram, L. (1995): Acetazolamide, benzodiazepines and lamotrigine. In *Typical absences and related epileptic syndromes*, eds J.S. Duncan & C.P. Panayiotopoulos, pp. 213–220. London: Churchill Livingstone.

Jeavons, P.M. (1977): Nosological problems of myoclonic epilepsies in childhood and adolescence. *Dev. Med. Child Neurol.* **19**, 3–8.

Manonmani, V. & Wallace, S.J. (1994). Epilepsy with myoclonic absences. *Arch. Dis. Child.* **70**, 288–290.

Panayiotopoulos, C.P., Ferrie, C.D., Knott, C., Robinson, R.O. (1993): Interaction of lamotrigine with sodium valproate. *Lancet* **341**, 445.

Richens, A. (1995): Ethosuximide and valproate. In *Typical absences and related epileptic syndromes*, eds J.S. Duncan & C.P. Panayiotopoulos, pp. 213–220. London: Churchill Livingstone.

Richens, A. & Yuen, A.W.C. (1991). Overview of the clinical efficacy of lamotrigine. *Epilepsia* **32** (Suppl 2), S13–S16.

Rowan, A.J., Meijer, J.W.A., de Beer-Pawlikowski, N. & van der Geest, P. (1983). Valproate-ethosuximide combination therapy for refractory absence seizures. *Arch. Neurol.* **40**, 797–802.

Sander, J.W.A.S., Hart, Y.M., Patsalos, P.N., Duncan, J.S. & Shorvon, S.D. (1991): Lamotrigine and generalized seizures. *Epilepsia* **32**, (suppl 1) S59.

Schlumberger, E., Chavez, F., Palacios, L., Rey, E. & Dulac, O. (1994). Lamotrigine in treatment of 120 children with epilepsy. *Epilepsia* **35**, 359–367.

Timmings, P.L. & Richens, A. (1992). Lamotrigine in primary generalized epilepsy. *Lancet* **339**, 1300–1301.

Subject Index